'Namaste Care seeks to engage peopl sensory input, especially touch, to becoming well established in the care] book by Nicola Kendall offers a stron̲g ----- , Namaste can be delivered to people with advanced dementia living in their own home, by engaging volunteers and family members in its delivery. This book not only details their experiences and the compassion that has been a driver for the service, but is also one that helps the reader to deliver Namaste Care themselves. This is a book I would recommend for family carers, as well as services who wish to embrace this sensitive and innovative care approach.'

– Dr Karen Harrison Dening, Head of Research and Publications, Dementia UK

'This informative and thought-provoking book is packed with helpful guidance in supporting people to live well with advanced dementia. It is a must-read for those who are working in care services and for those who are caring for individuals at home.'

– Jackie Pool, Director of Memory Care, Sunrise Senior Living UK

'More than a practical guide, this is a brilliant resource on Namaste Care – well written and insightful, providing a wealth of information. I recommend it wholeheartedly to anyone interested in Namaste Care. A timely publication given the rise in dementia, and the need to harness compassion in our communities.'

– Colette O'Driscoll, Namaste Care Manager, St Joseph's Hospice

'At a time when funding in health and social care is drastically reduced and the numbers of people living longer with dementia are increasing, this is an informed and inspiring handbook on how to address some of these issues. Training and building resilient communities is the key to allaying the fears around communicating with people with dementia, and supporting carers who have often fallen through the net of care. I know this approach works, through St Joseph's Hospice I set up the first Namaste Care Service in the UK which involved home visits – it's difficult, a balance of risk but one of the most rewarding projects I have worked on. If you are interested in setting up a similar service, this book will give you the impetus, confidence and insight and leave a lasting impact on you and your community.'

– Lourdes Colclough, former Namaste Care Manager,
St Joseph's Hospice, now Macmillan Engagement Manager

'A thorough and accessible guide. The subject is brought to life throughout with personal stories of how people living with advanced dementia can be supported to engage with the world and experience joy.'

– Isabelle Latham, Senior Lecturer, Association for
Dementia Studies, University of Worcester

Namaste Care for People Living with Advanced Dementia

of related interest

Visiting the Memory Café and other Dementia Care Activities
Evidence-based Interventions for Care Homes
Edited by Caroline Baker and Jason Corrigan-Charlesworth
ISBN 978 1 78592 252 7
eISBN 978 1 78450 535 6

Adaptive Interaction and Dementia
How to Communicate without Speech
Dr Maggie Ellis and Professor Arlene Astell
Illustrated by Suzanne Scott
ISBN 978 1 78592 197 1
eISBN 978 1 78450 471 7

Embracing Touch in Dementia Care
A Person-Centred Approach to Touch and Relationships
Luke Tanner
Foreword by Danuta Lipinska
ISBN 978 1 78592 109 4
eISBN 978 1 78450 373 4

Enhancing Health and Wellbeing in Dementia
A Person-Centred Integrated Care Approach
Dr Shibley Rahman
Forewords by Professor Sube Banerjee and Lisa Rodrigues
Afterword by Lucy Frost
ISBN 978 1 78592 037 0
eISBN 978 1 78450 291 1

Living Better with Dementia
Good Practice and Innovation for the Future
Shibley Rahman
Forewords by Kate Swaffer, Chris Roberts and Beth Britton
ISBN 978 1 84905 600 7
eISBN 978 1 78450 062 7

End of Life Care for People with Dementia
A Person-Centred Approach
Laura Middleton-Green, Jane Chatterjee, Sarah Russell and Murna Downs
ISBN 978 1 84905 047 0
eISBN 978 0 85700 512 0

Namaste Care for People Living with Advanced Dementia

A Practical Guide for Carers and Professionals

NICOLA KENDALL

With contributions from Joanne Atkinson, Barbara Edwards,
Chris Hayday, Lisa Howarth, Dr Caroline Jeffery,
Sharron Tolman, Ann White, Dr Trish Winter and Julie Young

FOREWORD BY **JOYCE SIMARD**

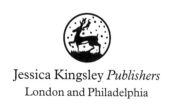

Jessica Kingsley *Publishers*
London and Philadelphia

Table 4.1 on page 40 is reproduced in amended format from Reisberg *et al.* 1982 with
kind permission from Barry Reisberg, M.D. Copyright © 1983 Barry Reisberg, M.D.
Table 4.2 on page 42 is reproduced in amended format from Reisberg 1984 with kind
permission from Barry Reisberg M.D. Copyright © 1984 by Barry Reisberg, M.D.
Figure 10.1 on page 84 is reproduced from James and Stephenson
2007 with kind permission from Ian A. James.
Figure 10.4 on page 89 has been adapted from Pearce 1999 and acknowledged as
developed by Northumberland Tyne and Wear NHS Foundation Trust.
The epigraph on page 113 is reproduced from Simard 2013
with kind permission from Joyce Simard.

First published in 2020
by Jessica Kingsley Publishers
73 Collier Street
London N1 9BE, UK
and
400 Market Street, Suite 400
Philadelphia, PA 19106, USA

www.jkp.com

Copyright © Nicola Kendall 2020
Foreword copyright © Joyce Simard 2020

Library of Congress Cataloging in Publication Data
A CIP catalog record for this book is available from the Library of Congress

British Library Cataloguing in Publication Data
A CIP catalogue record for this book is available from the British Library

ISBN 978 1 78592 834 5
eISBN 978 1 78450 975 0

Printed and bound in Great Britain

The accompanying PDF can be downloaded from www.jkp.com/catalogue/book/9781785928345

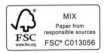

This book is dedicated to my beautiful Dorothy, who has taught me the true meaning of Namaste, and to Ernie Malt, who is a member of the Namaste Care Project steering group, and is an inspirational example of approaching a diagnosis of dementia with positivity and determination. Most importantly, this book has become about learning from and supporting my dad; my stubborn, determined, lovely dad, who is living with Lewy body dementia.

Contents

Foreword

Nicola Kendall has written this delightful book, *Namaste Care for People Living with Advanced Dementia*, that provides excellent, easy-to-follow ideas on implementing Namaste Care in a variety of settings.

I developed Namaste Care to help people with advanced dementia live with quality of life until the end of their life. The case studies included in this book show how professional and family carers can communicate in creative and meaningful ways with people who are living with advanced dementia.

I chose the name Namaste when I read that it meant 'to honour the spirit within', and this book is about the various ways carers touch the hearts of those who have difficulty communicating, thus honouring them and the life they have lived. Most of what is written about Alzheimer's disease is negative and hopeless. There are no medications that will stop the progression of an irreversible dementia, no cure on the horizon. Namaste Care shows how, in spite of the many losses people with dementia live with, they can still have pleasurable experiences. Family and professional carers will find so many ways to touch the hearts of the people they care for, and when they do, their hearts are also touched.

Joyce Simard

Acknowledgements

This book became a reality due to a combination of happy circumstances which I can only attempt to capture and acknowledge. Firstly, thanks are due to Andrew James, senior commissioning editor at Jessica Kingsley Publishers, who spotted my poster presentation about the Namaste Care Project at the Dementia Congress in Doncaster in 2017 and recognised the potential for a book on the subject. The kind input from editorial assistant Emma Scriver, production editor Claire Robinson, copyeditor Peter Dillon-Hooper and proofreader Colin Wood has been supportive and constructive in shaping this book into the final product.

St Cuthbert's Hospice senior management and trustees were the catalyst in recognising the need for this project when it was identified as a gap in services by the then Admiral Nurse, Sharron Tolman. The drive within the hospice is for continued development and achieving and maintaining excellence in services. I am incredibly fortunate to call the hospice my workplace.

Thanks must go to our funders, without whom the project, and so the book, would not have been possible. The initial funders who believed in the importance of improving care for people living with advanced dementia were the Albert Trust, the Rayne Foundation and the February Foundation. Bridge funding from February Foundation and the Ballinger Trust enabled the project to continue until we were amazingly fortunate to gain the three years Big Lottery Reaching Communities funding.

The amazing contributors, Joyce Simard, Trish Winter, Sharron Tolman, Lisa Howarth, Ann White, Barbara Edwards, Julie Young, Chris Hayday, Joanne Atkinson and Caroline Jeffery, have been incredible and generous in taking the time to write their respective pieces in the hope they can help families at an incredibly stressful time to step into their loved one's reality, and make every day count.

And finally, the support and absolute belief in me that I have had from my friends, family, volunteers and work colleagues has made the writing process a positive one and I am grateful for everyone who has encouraged me and given me feedback.

Nicola Kendall

1

Introduction

(including a case study contribution
from Dr Trish Winter, family carer)

At the Marie Curie Palliative Care Conference in 2017, a metaphor was used in one of the presentations which made a strong impact on the audience because it so accurately described the current mood within UK health services. Professor Max Watson from Hospice UK showed us a film he had taken on a recent trip to Niagara Falls. The huge volume of thundering water raced past, and in the distance the little *Maid of the Mist* boat made its tentative way forward, dwarfed by the falls. The *Maid of the Mist*, Professor Watson explained, reminded him of the National Health Service (NHS) at the moment, and the great deluge of water rushing towards it was the increasing and overwhelming level of need. The NHS is struggling against the current, and with resources being trimmed, rationalised and otherwise cut, this was how it would be for the foreseeable future.

What emerged from successive presentations at the conference that day was our need to enhance and strengthen the informal, unpaid care that exists within communities, and for professionals to become facilitators and co-ordinators of care, rather than necessarily being providers and directors of that care.

Added to this, the stark reality of dementia research was also brought into sharp focus by a summary article in *New Scientist* (Wise 2018). The article reflects on the regular media excitement at the prospect of a cure for dementia, where further stages in the drugs trials then prove to be ineffective failures. 'The disheartening reality is that there has been no new drug for dementia in fifteen years,' the article depressingly highlights. It would be easy to sink into gloom, in the face of what can appear to be insurmountable odds.

This book is therefore intended in a small way to redress the balance and give some hope that there are things that can be done to help. It is intended for family carers of people living with dementia, as well as professionals and paid carers. Given the growth of numbers of people being diagnosed with dementia globally, and with the lack of any hope for a cure any time soon, the focus must rest very firmly on ensuring the best possible care and quality of life for people diagnosed with dementia. According to the Dementia Statistics Hub, the current estimate of people living with dementia globally is 50 million, but this is expected to grow substantially to an estimated 152 million by 2050.[1] It is a widely feared and misunderstood condition. When I ask people in training or during presentations what words or phrases come to mind when they think of dementia, the most common answers are:

Memory loss

Confusion

Agitation

Getting lost

Forgetting

A living death

Deteriorating

While it would be wrong to pretend that all of these associations are untrue, I would take issue with one in particular: *a living death*. I hope within these pages to explore how we can change this view into something more positive. We can do this by understanding the changing needs of a person as their dementia progresses and by entering their reality, not expecting them to continue to fit into ours. In this way, we can also begin to use other words to describe the experience of dementia differently:

Connected

Engaged

Creative

Respectful

Emotional

---

1   www.dementiastatistics.org/statistics/global-prevalence

Joyful

A celebration of life

So, let me set the tone for the rest of the book by explaining the use of a very powerful word:

Namaste

Namaste means literally 'I bow to you' and is accompanied by a gesture of palms together over the heart and a bow of the head. It is a greeting and a parting in many cultures, and is used by Hindus, Muslims, Buddhists, Sikhs and in other religions, as well as in meditation, yoga and Reiki practice. However, it has a deeper symbolic meaning beyond being a mere greeting, which makes it very relevant to really 'seeing' the whole of the person with advanced dementia – acknowledging the *essence of who they are*. Often described as meaning 'honouring the spirit within', a further interpretation is 'the spirit within me honours the spirit within you'. This conveys a sense of equality, as the spirit within us is the same, and therefore a respectful, deep connection, which is beyond words or communication difficulties, is possible between two human beings. We can use different words for spirit, depending on our beliefs: soul, energy, divine spark, eternal self, atman, awen. What we mean is the spiritual part of us that is the core of who we are.

My favourite explanation of *namaste* takes this idea of spiritual connection even further:

Namaste
I honour the place within you in which the entire universe dwells.
I honour the place in you which is of love, of truth, of light and of peace.
When you are in that place in you and I am in that place in me,
We are one.

In the context of this book, I would also like to add my own words:

Dementia cannot touch this place, because this place
within you is pure, sacred and unchanging.

This may well sound very 'new age' and flowery to some readers, but approaching someone with advanced dementia with an open heart and a willingness to connect is the foundation on which we will build the Namaste Care approach described in this book.

Indeed, it was the word *namaste* that led me to my current job role as Namaste Lead at St Cuthbert's Hospice in Durham. In late 2016, I was looking online for a part-time job that might be suitable for my daughter while she was studying for her A-levels. To be fair, the 'Namaste Lead' job title did stand out as unusual amongst the other, more standard part-time job adverts for retail and domiciliary care. I think most people would have been intrigued by the job title, and so I clicked on it to find out more.

As I read down the job description and person specification, the list of mental ticks against each one led to a growing sense of excitement at this potential opportunity. Other than having very little dementia experience and not being trained in Namaste Care, I fitted all the other criteria, given my background in health and social care and in mental health. At the time, I was not actively looking for a new job, but something about this role strongly appealed. It involved setting up a new project from scratch, the funding was time limited and it was fewer hours than I was used to, but it felt like a very exciting way to bring together lots of strands of my previous experience. I was over the moon to be offered an interview and then to be offered the post, and I can say without hesitation that it is the most rewarding role I have had in my entire career.

It has been a steep learning curve, but more than two years on now the project is well established and recognised for the good work it delivers. I have a group of gorgeous volunteers who visit people with advanced dementia at home to share some Namaste Care with them, and we are generating some memorable, magic moments, some of which I will share in case studies in this book.

What has shocked me most about visiting the families at home for the first time and finding out their situation has been how much they struggle on with very little input from statutory services. I see spouses supporting their partners, despite having serious health issues themselves. I see social isolation, given that the children and grandchildren within a family are often working full time and unable to help or visit as much as they would like. In this context, a weekly visit from a volunteer is a true ray of sunshine, and the significance of that visit to the person with dementia, but also to their carer, should not be underestimated. As one husband told me, 'I don't feel on my own with her any more.'

However, Namaste Care is also a way that families can continue to connect with their loved one as the dementia progresses. I often hear people talk about a 'double loss' with dementia, in that it feels like the person is lost to the dementia even though they are still alive, and then they die and the loss hits again. Namaste Care cannot reverse the process of dementia, but it can provide special moments of connection and recognition that highlight that the person we love is still there, just harder to reach. Let me give you an example, by introducing you to my grandfather.

Grandad was a difficult man. That had nothing to do with his dementia. He was also a war hero and a respected policeman and always enjoyed being around children. He was never formally diagnosed with dementia, but for about the last six months of his life while he was living in a care home he had symptoms that I would now say were possibly vascular dementia. He would say and do inappropriate things to care staff, his language was confused and his memory of recent events was non-existent. I thought I was doing the right thing by keeping my young children away from him, as I feared what he might say. He was in and out of hospital with infections and his health deteriorated rapidly.

When he still lived at home, it had given him great joy to have visits from me and my children, who were four and seven at the time. He always offered the children grapes from his fruit bowl, and this became a little family ritual. I finally decided to chance taking them in to see him in the care home, given how ill he had been. Their presence was a trigger for a very lovely visit that I had with him, which proved to be the last time I would see him before he died.

As soon as he saw the children, he offered them grapes, as per the ritual. The thing was, he had no grapes in his room – the grapes he was offering out were invisible. Instinctively the children just went along with this, took the invisible grapes from him and pretended to eat them. During the entire visit, he did not say anything inappropriate. His face was lit up with delight at seeing the children and they were very natural with him in return. The children had evoked in him the recognition of a family ritual that had been important to him. The children holding his hand and chatting to him had lifted his spirits, and for a brief time, he was the Granda Tom that the children remembered.

What I see happening when people get to the stage of advanced dementia is a concentration on really good physical care, and it is good that people's physical needs are being well met. However, what I want to show you is that their need for stimulation mentally, emotionally and spiritually also continues at this time. If we set aside our preconceptions and experiment with different sensory approaches, based on what they have been interested in throughout their life, we can improve their quality of life greatly. Carers want to do the right thing (and often doubt their own abilities), and so Namaste Care provides an easy-to-learn and gentle framework through which you can enhance the time you have left with the person with dementia.

This time will be bittersweet without a doubt, but it has the potential to be meaningful and to allow you to maintain a positive relationship with the person you care for, until the end of their life. If you need any further convincing to read on, I'd like you to listen to the words of a loving daughter, Trish Winter, whose mum had Namaste Care visits from our volunteer Rosie.

I open the front door and my mum's head appears at the far end of the kitchen as she peers around the corner to investigate the sound. When she sees me her face breaks into a smile and she comes towards me with her arms outstretched. Her trousers are rolled up, her hair is dishevelled, she's happy and animated. Grabbing my hands, she leads me into the back room where I find Rosie sitting in one of the two reclining chairs. Rosie is surrounded by stuff. There are books, photographs, sheets of paper with poetry on them, Mum's treasured life-history book, towels, oils, lotion and a washing-up bowl full of water. The room is in disarray but the atmosphere is calm, purposeful and fragrant. This is the Namaste Care space that Rosie and Mum created together and that, in that moment, Mum was so keen to share with me.

In the years that Mum was living with dementia we encountered lots of different medical and care services, activities and groups. Some of these activities she enjoyed, some she tolerated and others she firmly refused to entertain. We heard much talk about 'person-centred care', but often these services, whilst well meaning, were not so person-centred in practice for reasons of resources, training or understanding. Mum had an unwavering radar for this and she fiercely exercised her power of refusal when something wasn't right for her. The Namaste Care approach, in our experience, was genuinely centred on Mum as a person, and this is why it was so powerful.

My mum had a great sense of fun, even in her darkest days. Shortly after she was admitted to hospital in what would be the final weeks of her life, she was taken for an X-ray. We wheeled along the corridor in a little cortege, Mum centre stage in a wheelchair pushed by a nurse with another nurse as side runner holding the bag of intravenous fluids aloft, and me bringing up the rear. We were approached by an oncoming cortege proceeding in the opposite direction. As we glided past each other, Mum acknowledged the crossing with a silent and stately thumbs up. When I later collected her from the X-ray, the technician was still laughing – when the flash went off, Mum had smiled for the camera. When Namaste Care talks of 'honouring the spirit', this is the spirit that I think of – the Mum whose humanity and sense of fun shone through at the very moment that she was reduced to the status of a frail body in a hospital bed. The Mum that was clever and studious and sang to us. The photographer and teacher. The magnificent baker who iced her own wedding cake and supplied us with scones, sausage rolls and lemon meringue pie. This was the Mum that Rosie honoured.

It was never a case of Rosie 'doing something' to Mum, jollying her along or trying to persuade her to get involved in an activity that somebody thought would be good for her. Instead, she skilfully and sensitively created an environment and a warm relationship where activities emerged between them, always with Mum's interests as a starting point. Although words were increasingly failing her, Mum had the pleasure of communication with Rosie in many different ways: through touch, poetry and walking together; through looking at pictures and reading stories of her life and her home town of Birtley; through songs, laughing and knitting. This communication and this relationship were built slowly over a period of time and they were real and meaningful.

Some of their activities re-ignited skills and interests that we thought had disappeared. A scarf was collaboratively knitted, with Mum's eagle eye monitoring and pointing out when Rosie had dropped a stitch. Perhaps the most significant event involved baking. One of the early signs of Mum's dementia was, in fact, that she started to forget how to do things in the kitchen. We started to realise that there were no more scones. Her signature chocolate cake, whose recipe was in her head, was no longer on the table. Losing the ability to bake must have been awful for her, and a shocking loss of identity. It's not surprising, then, that previous attempts by the family and others to support her with baking in the kitchen were met with stubborn refusal. Indeed, why would she want to go there again just to be reminded of what she could no longer do? Rosie knew about Mum's baking expertise but she didn't push it. She just patiently waited until the time was right. Then one day it was, and they baked together. I wasn't there, but my dad took photos and the expression on Mum's face says it all. Agreeing to bake with Rosie was the highest compliment that Mum could have paid her. And one that was extended to no one else, not even to members of the family.

The memory that I described in the first paragraph has become one of my most treasured memories from my mum's later life. As I replay it, I'm reminded that Namaste Care was not only important for Mum but for me and the family too. We feel privileged to have had Rosie and Namaste Care in our lives as well as in the life of our creative, sharp, skilled and fun-loving mum.

Each of the following chapters is intended as a guide based on experience of what needs to be considered as dementia progresses. The book describes what we have learned from our project, and so could be used to set up similar projects, or to incorporate the Namaste Care skills into existing projects, such as where befrienders already visit people with dementia. But I especially hope that it empowers family carers, given the incredible care they are giving in very difficult and stressful circumstances.

In 2014, a group of world experts from 23 countries agreed that the following areas were key in considering the palliative care needs of people living with dementia (van der Steen *et al.* 2014):

- Person-centred care

- Communication and shared decision-making

- Optimal treatment of symptoms and providing comfort

- Setting care goals and advanced planning

- Continuity of care

- Psychosocial and spiritual support

- Family care and involvement

- Education of the health care team

- Societal and ethical issues

I therefore thought it was important to extend the scope of the book to include guidance from experts about some of these elements, as they will enhance and support the Namaste Care approach.

In Chapter 2, we will explore in more detail what exactly Namaste Care is and the core elements that make up this gentle, sensory approach. I have asked Sharron Tolman to describe in Chapter 3 how her role as an Admiral Nurse led her to identify the need for the Namaste Care Project from her experience of what she saw families struggling with as dementia progressed. In Chapter 4, Lisa Howarth will clarify issues relating to identifying advanced dementia more specifically, to give us an understanding of the needs of people living with dementia at this time. In Chapter 5, we address dementia from a community perspective and discuss how to enhance the kindness that exists there. Moving on through the chapters we will look at the importance of the volunteer role, issues around the initial assessment, creating Life Stories and the psychological needs of the person living with dementia. A crucial issue that worries many carers is covered by Julie Young in Chapter 10, which is how to support people whose behaviour has changed.

Given the central role of the carer in supporting the person living with dementia, Chapter 11 then focuses on the support that they themselves require in order to continue with their vital role. We then go on to look in more detail at some key aspects of Namaste Care: sensory stimulation, loving touch and communication. The book also covers practical issues around the structuring of a Namaste Care session as well as reflecting on key learning so far gained from the project evaluations, including case study examples of people who have benefited from Namaste Care. The difficult but necessary topic of approaching end of life is discussed by Joanne Atkinson and Caroline Jeffery in Chapter 17.

In order to assist anyone setting up a Namaste Care Project, I have shared some resources within the Appendix that may serve as a starting point for establishing the administrative framework required. These forms are also available on the JKP website in downloadable format.

I also feel strongly that the Namaste Care approach does not need to be limited to use with dementia. I recognise many of the techniques, given my past experience working with people who have profound and multiple disabilities, and this approach would also translate to most medical conditions requiring palliative care.

A final word, before we get started. I have learned this the hard way. Whatever kind of carer that you are, you are a precious resource. It is not selfish to look after yourself. Indeed it is a necessary investment so that you can continue to do what you do. Consider always what you need for your own self-care, alongside what you are about to learn about caring for others. There will be more on this in Chapter 11, as it is so important to how a carer experiences the dementia journey alongside the person they care for. I hope in some small way that the book assists that journey.

2

What Is Namaste Care?

Joyce Simard, who is the creator of the Namaste Care Programme, is an incredibly inspirational speaker and writer. She will tell you herself that Namaste Care is not rocket science, but then she will say, with a smile, that she is not a rocket scientist. What is special about Namaste Care is that it comes at that time when people with advanced dementia may be receiving a good standard of physical care, as explained in the Introduction, but their ongoing need for meaning and stimulation is often overlooked. I often hear from family carers, when I make an initial visit to explain the project, things like:

'I really think you will be wasting your time.'

'Well, you can give it a go, but I don't think you'll get much response.'

'I'm worried that there are other people who you can be more help to. He/she is too far gone.'

So let's explain a little more about what exactly Namaste Care is:

Namaste Care is a gentle, sensory approach which focuses on engaging with someone living with advanced dementia through sound, touch, smell, taste and sight, in order to improve their quality of life as they approach the end of their life.

The first thing I will say is that you don't need to be an expert in dementia. I certainly wasn't when I took on the role, and many of our volunteers have never been around someone with dementia. What you do need is empathy, the ability to step into the shoes of another person and imagine how life is for them. We will however explore some issues that are of relevance to advanced dementia throughout the book as a way to reinforce a better holistic care approach.

Joyce Simard is a qualified social worker who worked in care homes in the USA and saw the accepted approaches to care for people with dementia in the early days of her career, with the priority being placed on attending to physical needs, but medicating or using various means of restraint to deal with wandering and agitated residents. This approach sees the person with dementia as 'a problem' to be solved, with the aim to 'keep them quiet'. She began first to develop groups for people with less advanced symptoms to keep them engaged and occupied. 'The Club' was a great success, but it still did not address the needs of people with advanced dementia symptoms, so Joyce turned her attention to this neglected group and really began to look at their needs.

Joyce began to see the importance of a calm and tranquil atmosphere, an encouraging, positive way of speaking to each person, the importance of loving touch, as well as the use of smells and music. So, this sensory approach began to evolve and grow. It became clear that the approach could be tailored to each person's likes and dislikes, and to what has been important in their lives. Finding the things that matter to each person is the key to open them up to experiencing some moments of connection and joy.

Let me summarise the core elements of Namaste Care as detailed by Joyce Simard, but also the key issues we have found to be important for delivering Namaste Care in a home setting, and then we can look at each in more detail.

- A person-centred approach
- Explaining the approach to the family and gaining their active support
- Completing a Life Story prior to starting sessions
- Addressing issues around comfort and pain management
- Creating a calming, peaceful and familiar environment for Namaste Care
- Use of a room spritz or aroma diffuser to scent the room
- Music playing which is meaningful to the person
- Natural use of loving touch, such as hand and foot massages, applying face creams or brushing hair
- Celebrating the seasons – bringing the outdoors inside

- Reminiscence activities such as memory boxes and photo albums

- Offering drinks throughout the session and sharing a favourite snack or treat

- Encouraging the person's range of movement

- Having fun!

- Feeding back to the family member or carer, and ideally involving them in sessions

We begin by exploring the contrast between the Namaste Care approach as it was originally designed for a care home environment and how it can be adapted to the home setting.

In the care home

Within a care home or inpatient setting where Namaste Care is offered, there is a Namaste room or area that can be adapted for use by a small group of residents with advanced dementia. Namaste Care happens for two hours in the morning and two hours in the afternoon. So once the resident has finished breakfast or lunch and has had their personal care needs attended to, they will be moved into the Namaste area. The room will already have been set up with subdued lighting, scents and music, so that people arrive into this calming atmosphere.

A member of staff greets each person as they arrive, settles them into the room and tucks them into their comfy chair with a cosy blanket. Each person has a drawstring bag with their name on, containing their personal items, such as their own hair brush, face cream and anything else specific to them. One or two members of staff can then spend time with each person within the group. At the end of the session, the worker can make notes about what was tried and any responses.

St Christopher's Hospice in London was the first organisation in the UK to introduce Namaste Care training for care home. With funding gained for a research project, a nurse researcher called Min Stacpoole led an evaluation of Namaste Care across five nursing homes in London. This resulted in some important key findings and the production of a 'toolkit' for anyone wishing to set up a Namaste Care project in a care home or inpatient setting (Stacpoole, Thompsell and Hockley 2016). It also contains valuable lessons learned about the importance of staff commitment to the success of the programme.

The most notable outcomes from the research carried out by St Christopher's and by research from the University of Western Sydney were that Namaste Care:

- reduced resident agitation and lethargy

- reduced the incidence of falls

- reduced urinary tract infections

- increased feeling of usefulness by family when they visited

- increased morale and job satisfaction for staff.

This improvement in the quality of life for people with advanced dementia can't be dismissed. The outcomes speak for themselves. At a time when family are stressed and deeply saddened by the progress of a brutal illness, the sight of a peaceful, happy member of their family who has just spoken or smiled for the first time in months is worth more than anything money can buy.

St Joseph's Hospice in Hackney, London, took the innovative step of introducing Namaste Care as a community project, whereby trained volunteers visit people with advanced dementia at home to share some Namaste Care activities. This is the model we adopted for our project at St Cuthbert's Hospice in Durham, although it is an ever-evolving project as we continue to learn lessons as we go along. Indeed the St Joseph's Hospice project has evolved by making links into a local hospital, providing Namaste Care by trained volunteers on the wards whilst people with advanced dementia are in hospital, and continuing this support on discharge. There are numerous benefits: it relieves pressure on nursing staff, identifies individuals who would benefit from Namaste Care, demonstrates the success of a more personal, sensory approach to medical staff and allows for a more linked-up network of support to surround the person.

The home environment

There are obvious contrasts between Namaste Care in an inpatient setting and in the person's own home. We have to work with what we've got in terms of an environment, but the home surroundings are familiar to the person and this seems to put people at ease. We are able to provide one consistent visitor, so this enables a lovely relationship to develop, both with the person with dementia and the family carer, who will often say they also look forward to the visits. Home visits also allow for more prolonged one-to-one attention, as compared to sharing the attention of a worker in a group within a care home. However, we do just visit once a week for up to two hours, so in comparison to four hours per day every day in a care home, the input is much reduced in terms of quantity, but certainly not in terms of quality.

Despite the shift to a community focus, we are just as true to the core elements of Namaste Care summarised previously, and so I will explore them now in a bit more detail.

A person-centred approach

Care services now recognise the importance of a person-centred approach as an accepted standard. However, within a care home or inpatient environment of rotas, staff shortages and turnover, groups with mixed needs and the pressure of numbers means that putting the person with dementia at the centre of all that you do and truly personalising their care can be a real challenge despite the best of intentions.

While the person living with dementia remains at home, this offers a much better opportunity to meet their needs in an entirely person-centred way. We will explore in much more detail the importance of person-centred planning in Chapter 8, when thinking about how Life Story work can inform the activities we might try with each person.

Explaining the approach to the family and gaining their active support

The success of visits is very much decided by how supportive the family is. I always begin by explaining what *namaste* means and why it was chosen to represent this particular programme. This seems to be a light bulb moment for families, and I explain that we will approach each visit with a 'let's try this and see what happens' frame of mind and that it is important for us to get to know what has been important to the person through a Life Story meeting. I also ensure that the family understands that volunteers have been police-checked, health-checked and fully trained, and are supervised, given that they are being asked to trust what is, at first, a stranger to enter their home and spend time with their loved one. Chapter 7 will describe in more detail this initial response to receiving a referral.

Completing a Life Story prior to starting sessions

Given the central importance of the Life Story in guiding how we will approach sessions, I have given this topic its own chapter (see Chapter 8). It is a humbling experience to facilitate the gathering of a Life Story and I am never bored by it. The Life Story is the foundation for the equality in the relationship between the person with dementia and their visitor. By understanding all that this person is and has been (child of someone, sibling of someone, partner, parent, worker, and so on), at a time when they may not be able to express or communicate their history themselves, allows us to deeply respect and honour this person's very essence and to assist them to continue to express who they are wherever possible.

Addressing issues around comfort and pain management

Put plainly, it is pointless to attempt activities that might improve someone's quality of life if they are sitting there in pain and discomfort. Lisa Howarth will discuss issues around the symptoms of advanced dementia in Chapter 4, and Julie Young also highlights the importance of recognising the person's needs in Chapter 10.

Family and carers often underestimate the pain that someone with advanced dementia may be in and can easily misread signs such as sitting quietly as meaning that there is not an issue with pain. Often at an advanced stage of dementia, the person is immobile and may have painful joints, be prone to pressure sores and rely on others to seat them in a comfortable position. It may be that a referral by the GP for a physiotherapy and occupational therapy assessment would be helpful to identify any equipment and exercises that would help. The GP can also advise on medication that might help the specific symptoms of the person with dementia.

Creating a calming, peaceful and familiar environment for Namaste Care

People relax when they feel safe, so this can be a guiding principle for us. What is it that would help this particular person to feel safe? It could be sitting in their favourite chair by the window, it could be that the family carer is in the next room, it could be a particular object. We will try to work this out in the initial visits or Life Story meeting.

Given that we are entering someone's home, we can't set up a room and greet the person into it. But we can adjust lighting, get the person comfortable, bring things nearer to them or take things with us to use in the session. Our own tone of voice and body language can also serve to calm and reassure, as well as explaining to the person what is going to happen next. This is discussed in more detail in later chapters.

Use of a room spritz or aroma diffuser to scent the room

A key part of creating the calm, relaxing atmosphere is the use of smells to scent the Namaste Care space. Joyce Simard advocates the use of lavender essential oils in a room spritz or diffuser, given that it has relaxing and gently sedative properties, which will also aid good-quality sleep. There is research to show the effectiveness of lavender in reducing agitation in people with advanced dementia (Holmes *et al.* 2002).

Another option we have tried is neroli oil (sweet orange), which is also relaxing but has the benefit of being an anti-depressant. The key thing is to keep the scent consistent, so that the person with dementia begins to associate the smell with a feeling of peace and relaxation; they may not remember each session, but they will remember the lovely feeling associated with Namaste Care. A few drops of essential oil added to water in a spray bottle or diffuser is all that is needed. Or you can purchase a hydrolat, which is the watery by-product from the distillation of the particular herb, and you can use this as the spritz.

One note of caution: it is always worth exploring (whether the person themselves can tell you or whether the family are aware of) any smells that might trigger a traumatic memory. Some examples of this include a lady who associated the smell of lemons with the death of a relative, the smell of smoke that reminded a man we worked with of an accident he had as a child, and a lady who linked the smell of floor polish to being punished as a child. The family are not always aware of these things, but it is worth finding out if possible.

Conversely, there may be a smell that invokes happy memories. The smell of rose for me means my lovely grandma, who made soft toys and crafts items and always added drops of rose perfume to the cushions she made. Her bedroom always smelled of roses too. In this, the sense of smell can be used in a positive way, either to help the person relax or to prompt recollections of times that will give them comfort. It is also worth considering continuing to use a favourite perfume or aftershave, as again this is a part of who this person is, and will be comforting for those close to the person as well as the person themselves. It's a sensory way of saying 'I'm still me'.

Music playing which is meaningful to the person

We will all have had the experience of being transported back to a teenage heartbreak by the music playing on the radio, or the sense of a certain time and place in our lives that hearing a particular piece of music reminds us of. Similar to our sense of smell, sound, and particularly music, is strongly associated with how memory is stored and seems to endure the progression of dementia much better than other forms of memory.

Quite simply, to honour who each person is, play the music that has been important to them in their lives and watch what happens. The lady that I visit at home, my very lovely Dorothy, loves Del Shannon. She even met him and shook hands with him after a concert when she was in her teens. This lady, who does not move independently any more, began moving her right arm in time to the music the first time I played her beloved Del Shannon to her. Reactions range from smiles, tapping along, humming and singing. Honestly, it's pure magic!

Natural use of loving touch, such as hand and foot massages, applying face creams or brushing hair

Touch appears to be an innate human need in all of us, and is an instinctive way to show comfort, reassurance and support. We naturally reach out to hold someone's hand or put an arm around them when they are distressed, and it has been shown that babies who are deprived of touch will fail to thrive and develop, and indeed may not survive. So, at a time when meeting physical care needs leads to a lot of functional, task-oriented touch, it is important to explore what other kinds of touch the person with dementia would benefit from.

Once again, the Life Story is vital. Not everyone is a 'touchy-feely' person and we need to be respectful of that. One family of a man I visited to complete a Life Story was very definite that a foot massage was not a good idea, as their dad had very ticklish feet and had once kicked out as a natural reflex at a nurse who had gone too near his feet; this man did like a hand massage though. So we can find out what makes sense to each person in terms of touch, whether it is having their fifties quiff hair style combed in, Pond's cold cream (also possibly Nivea, Astral, Oil of Olay or whatever the person's chosen face cream was) applied to the face as they always used to, or enjoying a relaxing hand massage with some scented hand cream or massage oil.

Many people we have worked with have also enjoyed having a twiddle mitt or sensory lap blanket to explore, as you will sometimes see people with advanced dementia picking at the material of their clothes and so on. Our local knitting groups have been enormously generous in their time (and wool). These too can be personalised, so an ex-professional footballer had a lap blanket in the colours of the club he played at, with bootlaces and other meaningful items added to make it unique to him.

Given the importance of loving touch, this will be discussed in more depth in Chapter 13, and guidance about massage will be suggested.

Celebrating the seasons – bringing the outdoors inside

Many people with advanced dementia will have the means to go outside, even once they are immobile, with equipment such as a wheelchair, hoist, adapted car and disabled ramp. However, from what I have seen in the community, it can be incredibly difficult in practice to do this regularly, especially when the main carer is a spouse who is also elderly and with health needs themselves.

Therefore, in order to help the person maintain a connection to the outdoors and to feel oriented to time and place, we can think of activities that are associated with the current season. From as simple as positioning the person so they can see out of a window, we can give some thought to what would help the person make sense of what is now for them. Taking in a box of dry leaves and pine cones in autumn, celebrating the various seasonal festivals relevant to their culture, reading poems about the season, filling a vase with seasonal flowers, having an ice cream on a hot summer day. Family and carers can have fun with this, and the fun will be catching.

One thing that we had not thought about when setting up the project was that not everyone with advanced dementia is immobile. Volunteers began to ask if it was okay to take the person they visited out for a walk. I checked with the insurers, and so long as a risk assessment was completed and signed by the carer, then yes, it was okay. So we have a small number of people who are still able to go out for a short walk near to where they live and to enjoy the birdsong and the budding trees in spring, and maybe have some interaction with neighbours or people that they pass by which they wouldn't have had otherwise. Obviously, each situation needs to be judged for safety and agreed with the family, but if it is possible, it's a lovely thing to do. At the very least, it may be possible to sit out in the garden or a park.

Reminiscence activities such as memory boxes and photo albums

Reminiscence is a common approach when working with people living with dementia. In practice, I would say yes, it's great, but it can cause problems too, so we need to be aware and sensitive to unexpected reactions.

One lady with early-onset dementia, who used to work as an administrator, enjoys mindful colouring and holds two different coloured pencils in one hand as she would have done for many years no doubt with pens. So, finding an activity that taps into a long-held skill is a lovely way to encourage the person to continue to express who they are. You will find a person able to play a guitar or the piano, long after you think they will have forgotten how.

Making memory boxes full of special, meaningful items, or looking through old photographs, can elicit conversation or recognition. Giving the person with dementia a lifelike baby doll or pet animal, if that was meaningful to them, can bring great pleasure and comfort.

However, we have found that it is also easy to make assumptions about such things and get it very wrong. I completed a Life Story of a lady who had worked in the legal profession and this relied a lot on what her husband was able to tell me. This lady has a type of dementia that affects her ability to express herself, but not her understanding of what is being said. I was very pleased with myself that I had a volunteer who shared this lady's interest in horses. I was sad to hear that after the Life Story visit, this lady had been very depressed for the following couple of weeks. When the volunteer visited, she very definitely did not want to look at old pictures of herself from when she used to ride her horse. What we realised was that, in our well-meaning but naïve way, we had reminded her of all the things she could not do or had lost. The volunteer found that connecting through massage and giving space for her to express her emotions was the key to building their relationship, not any kind of reminiscence approach.

We have also had situations where people with advanced dementia are not able to recognise the people in photographs, and this can be distressing to them and to the family witnessing this.

Offering drinks throughout the session and sharing a favourite snack or treat

At this stage of dementia, the person will most likely be dependent on others to prompt them to eat and drink. Hydration is very important in preventing urinary tract infections, chest infections and blood-clotting problems. When

Namaste Care was first introduced in a US care facility by Joyce Simard, they reported a dramatic decline in these kinds of infections. If there are any problems with swallowing and coughing, a speech and language therapist can carry out an assessment and may well recommend thickeners be added to the drink to reduce the issue of fluids entering the lungs (aspiration). So anyone visiting the person needs to be made aware of these requirements.

Often people in late-stage dementia lose interest in food as well. A Namaste Care session provides an opportunity to share something that the person would consider a treat, and due to the social nature of the interaction the person often seems more willing to eat. For some reason, at this stage the preference is often for sweet treats, but again adaptations may need to be made to accommodate eating difficulties. For example, if a person has always enjoyed chocolate but can no longer chew well, a chocolate mousse could be the thing to try.

This is a time when the family can be faced with making a best-interest decision on behalf of their loved one who may be having swallowing difficulties. An option would be a PEG tube, which involves an operation and a tube being inserted so that food or liquid can be given directly into the stomach. Many families make the decision not to have this procedure for their loved one, especially if that person really loved their food. It is an individual quality-of-life decision for the family to make in each case.

Encouraging the person's range of movement

We all know that if we sit for long periods of time, we become stiff and our joints can feel painful. So, if the person living with dementia is no longer mobile or able to move independently, we can help them gain some relief by changing positions regularly, but also by gently encouraging the range of movement on each joint. This can be done through a particular activity that encourages movement, such as reaching for something (active movement), or we may have to support the joint and gently move it through its range ourselves on behalf of the person (passive movement). Often the person may have arthritis with joints especially painful and swollen, so care must be taken to respect the person's expressions of pain or unwillingness to participate. Not forcing any movement, and ideally with the advice of a physiotherapist, this can really enhance a person's wellbeing and level of pain and discomfort; but always observe and respect non-verbal cues from the person.

Having fun!

Joyce Simard is keen to remind us that having dementia doesn't have to be all doom and gloom. Being able to raise a smile, and better still, a hearty laugh, is evidently beneficial to the wellbeing of the person living with dementia. Reading silly limericks, blowing bubbles, showing the person funny pictures and even getting dressed up in humorous costumes, silly hats, wigs and masks can all brighten a person's day. Joyce uses a cute dog hand puppet to entertain people, and this is much loved by the people she works with. On this theme, this is where our ego and self-consciousness need to be left at the door and we need to be prepared to go and be more free and child-like in how we express ourselves.

Feeding back to the family member or carer, and ideally involving them in sessions

As a visitor into a family home, I am always struck by the act of trust families make in opening their home to us. I take time to talk to the family at the beginning of each visit to find out how things are, providing some listening and empathy for what is a stressful role. Then at the end of each session, it is nice to take some time to explain what you have tried with their family member and what responses occurred.

We have found that some family carers use the time we visit as a mini respite from being on constant high alert, and that in itself is a real benefit. Given that it is a volunteer that is visiting, we ask for a carer to be present in the house, but they don't need to stay in the room.

Over time, family members often show more and more interest in what we are doing, and the reality is, given that they are with the person most of the time, their choosing to learn about Namaste Care would be ideal, so that they could use it on a daily basis.

As one daughter commented in the research carried out by St Christopher's Hospice in London:

> The biggest thing Namaste has given me is a different focus when visiting mum. For many years now mum hasn't been able to communicate with us and conversation has been one sided which is difficult and at times she appeared to barely realise I was there. I now know to do other things as well as talk to mum, like show her old photos, brush her hair, feed her treats, and moisturise her face and hands. This makes spending time with her easier

and I feel I'm making more of a connection with her and a difference in her life.[1]

Benefits for everyone

I hope this summary has given a flavour of what Namaste Care is and how to approach it. You will find it to be rewarding for the person living with dementia, the volunteer, the close and wider family, as well as any professionals involved, because it celebrates the life of this unique person, with all that makes them who they are. It can be continued right up to the person's death. I spent some very special and precious times with a lady who came into St Cuthbert's Hospice for end-of-life care, and in her final days, she still enjoyed a hand massage. She would sniff her hand afterwards and say, 'Ooo, that's lovely, pet.'

In the next chapter, Consultant Admiral Nurse Sharron Tolman will describe how her role as an Admiral Nurse led her to identify the need for the Namaste Care Project at St Cuthbert's Hospice in Durham. Sharron works for Dementia UK, which is an organisation that recognises the importance of the Namaste Care approach and which supported her to help me with establishing the Namaste Care Project at St Cuthbert's Hospice when she was the Admiral Nurse there (and my boss). It was her visits to support families that had identified the need for services for people living with advanced dementia, and Sharron spent two years trying to gain the initial funding for the Namaste Care Project.

I have a lot to thank her for, and I am thrilled that she is able to share some of her knowledge by contributing to this book.

---

1   Email from the daughter of a resident – quoted in the Namaste Care Toolkit (Stacpoole *et al.* 2016). Copyright © St Christopher's 2016.

3

Admiral Nursing and the Origins of the Namaste Care Project at St Cuthbert's Hospice

Sharron Tolman (Consultant Admiral Nurse, Dementia UK)

Admiral Nurses are registered nurses who have specialist knowledge of dementia care and provide support to family carers and people living with dementia throughout the trajectory of dementia, particularly during complex periods of transition. The aim of Admiral Nursing is to improve the wellbeing and quality of life of the person with dementia and their family carer and enhance their ability to adjust and cope with dementia. Admiral Nurses also enhance colleagues' knowledge and experience of working with people affected by dementia, through consultancy, leadership and education. Admiral Nurses use a family- and relationship-centred approach, working in partnership with families and colleagues to achieve best practice and positive outcomes. Admiral Nurses work in many areas of practice: community, care home, acute hospital, home care, hospices, clinics and the Admiral Nurse Helpline.

Admiral Nurses were named by the family of Joseph Levy CBE BEM, who founded the charity. Joseph had vascular dementia and was known affectionately as 'Admiral Joe' because of his love of sailing.

Dementia UK is a registered charity with a vision to provide specialist and compassionate dementia support for all families that need it and lead and deliver high-quality expert and accessible dementia care through Admiral Nursing. Dementia UK is committed to making a real difference to families living with the effects of dementia (Dementia UK 2017b).

St Cuthbert's Hospice, Durham, was the first hospice in the UK to appoint an Admiral Nurse, an innovative partnership with Dementia UK. With more and more people diagnosed with dementia, currently 850,000 people living with the condition in the UK (Alzheimer's Society 2014), it is essential to develop services that address the needs of those affected by more advanced dementia and at end of life.

Dementia is a life-limiting condition without curative treatments, but this is often still not recognised. It is the leading cause of death in England and Wales.[1] Earlier in dementia, when people have capacity it's important to consider and talk with family about what's important as the condition progresses: their preferences, values and needs regarding the future. Making decisions on behalf of the person with dementia can be particularly hard, so any information or guidance about people's preferences can help inform decisions. For example, asking: What if you became more ill? Where would you like to be cared for? What if you developed an infection, would you like to be admitted to hospital or have treatment at home? What do you think you, your family and friends would want to know if you became more unwell? If your condition worsens, what are your goals, fears? (Middleton-Green et al. 2017).

As things change and people approach end of life, understanding this progression, treatment options and maximisation of comfort are key goals of care. Common symptoms such as pain and constipation can be missed when behavioural change and distress are seen as symptoms of the dementia rather than the effects of those underlying causes. The dementia is often 'blamed'. Despite a preference for care at home at end of life (Poole et al. 2017), the number of people with dementia dying at home remains low, with most people dying in care homes. End-of-life care is recognised as the last 12 months of life (NICE 2011), but the course of dementia can be unpredictable, particularly as the person with dementia is likely to be living with other illnesses too. Observing for possible indicators – reduced function, more withdrawn, reduced communication and changes to eating and drinking – can help, or asking the 'surprise question': Would I be surprised if the person died within the next 6 to 12 months? (Gold Standards

---

1   www.ons.gov.uk/peoplepopulationandcommunity/birthsdeathsandmarriages/deaths/bulletins/deathsregisteredinenglandandwalesseriesdr/2017

Framework Centre 2016). Nevertheless, recognising end of life in dementia is complex, but planning ahead and considering the possibility of death at any time helps to avoid having to make difficult decisions at times of crisis or heightened distress.

Current estimates suggest 700,000 friends and family are caring for a person with dementia in the UK (Alzheimer's Research UK 2015). Family carers provide significant physical and emotional care as dementia progresses, which can impact negatively on their own health and wellbeing. In my community visits, I witnessed the lack of support for people in the late stages of dementia. Recognising the gap in provision for people in later stages of dementia and the need for people with dementia to have better end-of-life care experiences, St Cuthbert's Hospice sought to reach out to people with dementia who may be in the last years of life and still living at home with their family carer. We worked together with Hope for Home, to gain funding to set up the Namaste Care Project, initially for an 18-month pilot. Families often feel ill equipped or prepared for what may lie ahead, and so the project aimed to provide support for them also and a 'link' to the hospice should they need more specialist palliative care.

It was a huge pleasure to be part of setting up this service. The skills and compassion our volunteers demonstrate are beyond anything I ever imagined, and people with dementia and their families are benefiting from meaningful engagement at a time of their life when other services often say, 'There's nothing we can do, it's the progression of dementia.' Namaste Care offers hope that there is something we can do.

4

Advanced Dementia and Assessment

Lisa Howarth (Admiral Nurse, St Cuthbert's Hospice)

Advanced dementia is a complex area and is at times difficult to define. Dementia is a unique experience to the person living with it, and this is the same when the person progresses to the advanced stages. How and when the person reaches advanced dementia can be difficult to determine. Some people live well with moderate dementia for a significant time before the signs and symptoms of advancement or progression of dementia are seen. Other people can seem to enter the later stages quite rapidly in comparison, and there is no reasoning to this other than how the dementia affects that individual's brain throughout their time living with dementia.

Because of this complexity, it can be very difficult to assess people for Namaste Care. In this chapter I hope to explore issues to consider when someone is referred to the Namaste Care service. We will look at issues that have challenged us around inappropriate referrals, professional boundaries and managing expectations from the service.

The dementia journey

It feels appropriate to begin with thinking about whom Namaste Care is for and what guidance we give to those referring people into the service.

Joyce Simard (2013) founded the concept, and although this was initially intended for care homes, our Namaste Care Project reach was to connect to people in their own home, which in itself was difficult at first. Various articles about Namaste Care, including Thompsell, Stacpoole and Hockley (2014), have shown the positive results when using Namaste Care in care home environments, such as reduction in severity of neuropsychiatric symptoms like agitation and restlessness. Residents responded to the different elements of the intervention, such as massage and music, and were more alert and did interact more with others due to the calming and relaxing approach. This gave rewarding benefits as staff and family connected with the person receiving the care, and it encouraged creativity and increased confidence. The main outcome from Namaste Care was there was no evidence that it caused harm. So, our biggest task was to transfer this concept into people's own home on a one-to-one basis and to ensure similar results were achieved.

With people living in care homes who have a diagnosis of dementia, progression of symptoms may be noticed by family and carers and they have 24-hour support within that environment, and embedding Namaste Care in a familiar place with trained carers can be evaluated more readily. Our challenge was to seek out families and professionals involved in caring for people with advanced dementia who were still at home, often with families being main carers and/or with robust care packages.

Initially the Namaste Care service took the concept to pre-existing embedded dementia services, such as the Alzheimer's Society, community mental health teams, allied health professionals and carers support, to tell the community about the service and encouraged people to ask questions and refer to the service. This led to a vast variety of referrals, ranging from mild, newly diagnosed dementia, to moderate dementia, to some who were indeed in the more advanced stages.

When the initial referrals came in to the project, it became evident that people's definition of advanced dementia was hugely variable and there seemed confusion on when was best to refer to the service. As the referrals continued to come in to the Namaste Care Project, several challenges faced the Namaste Lead. These included, how do we ensure the right people are receiving the service? For those who weren't in the advanced stages, the project team felt a responsibility still to offer them something, as there was clearly an unmet need. It also raised issues about professional boundaries for the project and also managing expectations of what the families may want.

As mentioned, there are lots of issues to consider when assessing someone for Namaste Care, so to break this down I feel it may be appropriate to look at each section starting with the referral criteria.

Due to the variation in types of referrals, it seemed appropriate to create some referral guidelines, to help people when thinking about referring into the service and to ensure those appropriate for Namaste Care gained access to it. We looked at the literature about advanced dementia to start defining referral criteria.

We started by looking at the ongoing journey of dementia; health professionals sometimes discuss stages, which refers to how a person's dementia has progressed. This can help determine the best treatment approach, and these stages can be added to a scale. The Global Deterioration Scale (GDS) (Reisberg *et al.* 1982) divides the disease into seven stages based on the amount of cognitive decline (see Table 4.1).

Table 4.1: Global Deterioration Scale (GDS)

Diagnosis	Stage	Signs and symptoms	Expected duration of stage
No dementia	Stage 1: No cognitive decline	In this stage, the person functions normally, has no memory loss, and is mentally healthy. People with NO dementia would be considered Stage 1.	N/A
No dementia	Stage 2: Very mild cognitive decline	This stage is used to describe normal forgetfulness associated with ageing. For example, forgetting names and where familiar objects were left. Symptoms of dementia are not evident to the individual's loved ones or their physician.	Average duration of this stage is between 2 and 7 years
No dementia	Stage 3: Mild cognitive decline	This stage includes increased forgetfulness, slight difficulty concentrating and decreased work performance. People may get lost more frequently or have difficulty finding the right words. At this stage, a person's loved ones will begin to notice a cognitive decline.	Average duration of this stage is 2 years
Early stage	Stage 4: Moderate cognitive decline	This stage includes difficulty concentrating, decreased memory of recent events, and difficulty managing finances or travelling alone to new locations. People have trouble completing complex tasks efficiently or accurately and may be in denial about their symptoms. They may also start withdrawing from family or friends because socialisation becomes difficult. At this stage, a physician can detect clear cognitive problems during a patient interview and exam.	Average duration of this stage is 2 years

Mid-stage	Stage 5: Moderately severe cognitive decline	People in this stage have major memory deficiencies and need some assistance to complete their daily living activities (dressing, bathing, preparing meals, etc.). Memory loss is more prominent and may include major relevant aspects of current lives. For example, people might not remember their address or phone number and might not know the time or day or where they are.	Average duration of this stage is 1.5 years
Mid-stage	Stage 6: Severe cognitive decline (middle dementia)	People in Stage 6 require extensive assistance to carry out their activities of daily living (ADLs). They start to forget names of close family members and have little memory of recent events. Many people can remember only some of earlier life. Individuals also have difficulty counting down from 10 and finishing tasks. Incontinence (loss of bladder or bowel control) is a problem in this stage. Ability to speak declines. Personality/emotional changes, such as delusions (believing something to be true that is not), compulsions (repeating a simple behaviour, such as cleaning) or anxiety and agitation, may occur.	Average duration of this stage is 2.5 years
Late stage	Stage 7: Very severe cognitive decline (late dementia)	People in this stage have essentially no ability to speak or communicate. They require assistance with most activities (e.g. using the toilet, eating). They often lose psychomotor skills; for example, their ability to walk.	Average duration of this stage is 1.5 to 2.5 years

Namaste Care is predominantly aimed at people in Stage 7 of this model, although it could be argued that people in Stage 6 would also benefit.

Confusingly, someone could score badly on a cognitive test, such as the 6 Item Cognitive Impairment Test or the more detailed ACE III (Addenbrooke's Cognitive Examination-III), but still be functioning reasonably well. It is therefore also worth referrers looking at how a person is functioning. There is a Functional Assessment Staging Test (FAST) by Reisberg (1988), and this scale also looks at the seven stages but looks at functioning level and ability to perform daily living activities (see Table 4.2). A person may be at a different stage cognitively on the GDS stage than functionally on the FAST stage.

Table 4.2: Functional Assessment Staging Test (FAST)

Stage	Patient condition	Level of functional decline	Expected duration of stage
Stage 1	Normal adult	No functional decline	N/A
Stage 2	Normal older adult	Personal awareness of some functional decline	Unknown
Stage 3	Early Alzheimer's disease	Noticeable deficit in demanding job situations	Average duration of this stage is 7 years
Stage 4	Mild Alzheimer's	Requires assistance in complicated tasks such as handling finances, travelling, planning parties, etc.	Average duration of this stage is 2 years
Stage 5	Moderate Alzheimer's	Requires assistance in choosing proper clothing	Average duration of this stage is 1.5 years
Stage 6	Moderately severe Alzheimer's	Requires assistance with dressing, bathing and toileting; experiences urinary and faecal incontinence	Average duration of this stage is 3.5 months to 9.5 months
Stage 7	Severe Alzheimer's	Speech ability declines to about half a dozen intelligible words; progressive loss of ability to walk, to sit up, to smile and to hold head up	Average duration of this stage is 1 year to 1.5 years

Again, Namaste Care would be aimed at people in Stage 7. The people with dementia and their families who have refused the offer of Namaste Care tend to be people who have scored poorly on a cognitive test but who would score as moderate on a functional test. We would therefore advise that, as a general rule, a functional assessment can be a better indicator for Namaste Care than a cognitive assessment. However, we do have examples where this is the other way around, which highlights the individual nature of dementia.

We also encourage referrers, whether that be family or professionals, to think about how long the person has had dementia, and we also talk to the family about the dementia and cognitive decline, as collateral history is the key to getting the most accurate account of the patient's journey with dementia (Hughes 2011).

With these indicators in mind, the referral guidelines for the project were created and will be regularly reviewed as we continue to learn.

Namaste Care Project: Referral criteria guidance

Namaste Care was developed by Joyce Simard in the USA as an end-of-life programme for people living with advanced dementia. Whilst defining advanced dementia is quite difficult, given that individual symptoms differ, and progression of symptoms can be so varied, the following criteria are intended to provide guidance on appropriate referrals for the community-based Namaste Care Project.

- It would not surprise you if the person living with dementia is most likely in their last year of life.

- The person living with dementia is finding it more difficult to communicate verbally.

- They have become completely dependent on the support of others for activities of daily living.

- They would not now find it easy to leave the house or engage in group activities.

- They would benefit from a more gentle, sensory approach, on a one-to-one basis.

- The carer is aware that they need to be present in the house during Namaste visits by trained volunteers.

An issue that can be mistaken for progression of symptoms (and can indeed lead on to progression of symptoms) is if someone develops delirium. Symptoms of delirium can include increased confusion, disorientation, difficulties with concentration, hallucinations and behaviour changes. It is easy to see how these symptoms are difficult to recognise in someone with dementia who may already be experiencing some of these symptoms. The distinguishing feature of delirium is that it comes on very suddenly and is often caused by the person being physically unwell. Delirium is a treatable condition, but if it goes unrecognised and untreated it can be fatal in extreme cases.

A useful prompt for examining the underlying cause for the delirium is PINCHME:

- Pain

- Infection

- Nutrition

- Constipation

- Hydration

- Medication

- Environment

Medical professionals can use this guide to explore and treat the causes of delirium. 'In hospitals, approximately 20–30% of older people on medical wards will have delirium and up to 50% of people with dementia. Between 10–50% of people having surgery can develop delirium' (Dementia UK 2017a). Delirium, as well as dementia, will often lead to longer hospital stays and will increase the risk of falls, accidents, pressure sores and a care crisis. It is therefore important that everyone works even more closely together during this acute phase to support the person living with dementia and the family.

Challenges we faced

After looking more in-depth at what the literature says about advanced dementia and at how we created referral guidelines, it seemed appropriate to think about how we reached out to the families, carers and professionals who we want to refer into the services.

This was a sensitive area, as asking people to refer to the Namaste Care service involved getting people to think about their loved one's prognosis and potentially raise issues that they might not have considered previously, as their loved one may have subtly progressed to these advanced stages without anyone speaking of it or its being noticed. Ultimately it can focus people's thinking that possibly they had a limited amount of time left with their loved one, and this can be very difficult to acknowledge and process. This highlights the importance of regular review for people living with dementia to enable discussion of progression or changes (NICE 2018).

We have already learnt that it is difficult having end-of-life conversations, as discussed in 'Dying Matters',[1] and by the time people are needing Namaste

---

1   www.dyingmatters.org/page/Talkingaboutdeathdying

Care they may lack capacity (under the Mental Capacity Act 2005), and some have never had conversations about end of life before. By the time that the person reaches the advanced stages of dementia, it is often too late for these discussions.

We discovered that this area of dementia care was one that has little resource nationally, but it is acknowledged nationally as an area of great importance (as documented in Hospice UK 2015). Our project is innovative within our geographical area, and while people agreed it was needed and was an area to develop, it became clear that defining advanced dementia was difficult for professionals as well as families.

In the early stages, when the Namaste Care service was being set up, we did not have the clear direction and the guidelines that we later came to develop, and in a way the early referrals aided us to create these guidelines to ensure those who were in the advanced stages, for whom Namaste Care was designed, were referred to the service.

Once we received a referral, we made contact and arranged an initial appointment to meet the person living with dementia and discuss the interventions. At this first appointment a lot of information was given, and a lot of information received, about the person living with dementia. Some referrals were found to be not suitable for Namaste Care; this was for a variety of reasons, although the main one was that the person being referred was not in the advanced stages of dementia. But often it was clear there was an unmet need and that Namaste Care might benefit. In such cases the Namaste Lead felt a responsibility to do something to help and support the person and the family.

At St Cuthbert's Hospice these referrals were brought back and discussed with the Admiral Nurse. Sometimes it was clear that the family needed support, so the Admiral Nurse could become involved and offer support to the family. If the person met the criteria they were discussed with the Admiral Nurse, and some were referred for cognitive stimulation therapy at the hospice, which is a 14-week programme and has access to ongoing advice from the Admiral Nurse, or signposting to the Dementia Advisor Service run locally by the Alzheimer's Society, or alternatively community groups were offered to the person and families.

For the families who were supported within the Namaste Care Project, what was observed by the Lead and the volunteers was how isolated some of the families could be, with little social interaction week on week. Professionals such as district nurses, GPs and care agencies tended to be the main contact families received, as often friendships had faded away once the person living with dementia struggled in social situations and became housebound.

The Namaste Lead, in having matched the people concerned and being responsible for reviewing progress, as well as the volunteer visitors, all felt a deep sense of commitment to building a strong and enduring relationship that enhances the life of the person living with dementia. This would lead to the creation of volunteer supervision groups being developed to ensure that the volunteers had support and an opportunity to talk issues through with the Lead and Admiral Nurse and to ensure that the project had a support network that could discuss concerns, issues, positive experiences, and professional boundaries. This supervision was important to develop, as Nicola (author/Lead) and Barbara (volunteer) will discuss in other areas of the book; a close bond is formed between the volunteer, the person receiving Namaste Care and their families, and this needs to be supported and nurtured but also protected. Being able to live as well as possible with advanced dementia needs a multi-professional approach. The volunteer, support worker and Lead need to know when and where to access support, when changes are occurring or when more care/medical input is needed, to have trust in other services available and to understand that they are part of a network that supports the person living with advanced dementia.

This discussion about professional boundaries/clinical supervision follows neatly into managing expectations. As the volunteers build relationships with both the person living with dementia and their families, there are a great many positive aspects to being involved in Namaste Care, as Nicola will describe throughout this book. One area I feel needs further discussion is the managing of expectations.

The amazing interventions that the project witnesses, and the magic moments that we hear about in supervision, are testimony to the ongoing need to maintain and develop Namaste Care. There have been, at times, some expectations from families of their loved ones that prove to be challenging for those carrying out Namaste Care. For example, there have been times where families have desperately wanted the magic moments to happen while they are present or they feel they have not seen any change, or that with some one-on-one intervention their loved ones may talk again or regain a lost skill. This can be difficult for the families and the person carrying out the Namaste Care visit, as they don't want to feel they have created an unrealistic expectation. This is where the supervision has been paramount, so the volunteers can talk about this in a safe environment.

There is also the potential expectation that the volunteer is there to do other things to help the families such as collecting prescriptions, or helping out with phone calls. This may seem like small tasks, and some may think it would be okay to help the family with this. We do agree in some ways, but we need to be aware of creating dependency by the carer on the volunteer. We do encourage the carer to use the Namaste Care time for some respite for themselves, but we need to ensure that volunteers keep within the scope of the project and do not put themselves in any vulnerable situations. This is discussed with the Namaste Lead, volunteers, the person who is going to receive Namaste Care and the carer, when a meeting is held to introduce the volunteer to the person who is going to be receiving Namaste Care and the family. This discussion outlines what interventions may be performed during the sessions and expectations of the sessions and of the volunteer. It is at this point that a three-way agreement is signed to demonstrate this discussion has taken place and that all parties agree (see Appendix).

5

Harnessing Community Kindness

(with a contribution from Ann White MBE,
Dementia Friends Champion)

One of the consistent themes I hear from people when I first visit them is how friends and sometimes family have seemed to avoid contact once a person is diagnosed with dementia. Wendy Mitchell talks about this happening to her in her book *Somebody I Used to Know* (2018) and how she went about tackling the issue head on when she saw a neighbour deliberately avoiding speaking to her. What she found was a feeling of awkwardness people have and a sense of their not knowing what to say or what to expect. Added to the frequent experience of GPs seeming unable to know what to do and not having the time to support families through this, the situation makes for a very isolating and stressful experience. As Wendy Mitchell notes, 'I have heard nothing from any doctor since my diagnosis three months ago.'

However, dementia is a community issue, as I argued in the Introduction. I think there is a common misconception that people with dementia, especially in advanced stages, are being cared for in residential homes. The reality is that over 60 per cent of people are still living at home in the community[1] and being predominantly cared for by spouses, close family and some paid-for home care by care agencies.

Compassionate Communities UK is one response to the reality that, 95 per cent of the time, people will have no contact with health services and professionals.

---

1 www.dementiastatistics.org/statistics/care-services

Compassionate communities are communities that squarely recognize the major but under-recognized, the least spoken about, and the most overlooked human experiences in all communities – serious illness, ageing, dying, care giving and loss – and the need to recognize that even these populations have a right to health and wellbeing strategies to address the additional morbidities (illnesses) and mortalities (deaths) that are consequences of their other experiences of ageing, serious illness, care giving and loss.[2]

Compassionate Communities UK provides education programmes and consultancy and aims to guide policy at local, regional, national and international levels. One of the contributors to Compassionate Communities UK is Dr Julian Abel, who is a consultant in palliative care. He also spoke at the Marie Curie Palliative Care Conference in 2017. He wrote the guidance to Ambition 6 of the National End of Life Strategy: The End of Life Ambitions Framework 2015–2020. Ambition 6 is 'Communities are prepared to help'. Translating strategy and ambition into action takes a vision, and sometimes a small, humble vision such as Namaste Care might just be the focus that local people need to find an expression for the kindness and compassion that very clearly exists, but is drowned out by media stories of crime, intolerance and a consumer-driven culture.

So let's discuss compassion a little further.

Being compassionate

Compassion is a concept that is deeply embedded in our human consciousness. It may also prove to be crucial to our wellbeing in a world now shared by more than seven billion people. Indeed, the capacity for compassion in the human mind and heart, recently a topic of study in the neurosciences and the subject of ongoing discussions in psychology, ethics, literature and theology, may be key to the very survival of humankind as well as the environment we share with other creatures.[3]

Compassion is the concern and understanding for the difficult experiences of others. Its Latin root, *compati*, means to 'suffer with', and I have observed the suffering felt by family and carers in direct response to what they see as the suffering of the loved one with dementia. Neuroscientists have been examining the biological basis for compassion by measuring brain regions,

2   www.compassionate-communitiesuk.co.uk/what-we-do
3   https://charterforcompassion.org/index.php/being-compassionate

heart rate, levels of the bonding hormone 'oxytocin' and activity of the vagus nerve. The Greater Good Science Center at the University of California came up with the following definition of compassion as a result of these studies: '[Compassion] is defined as the feeling that arises when you are confronted with another's suffering and feel motivated to relieve that suffering.'[4]

Whilst there are active campaigns to encourage people not to use the phrase 'suffering with dementia' in order to create a more positive view that it is possible to live well with dementia, the fact that witnessing the disease progression of someone living with dementia creates compassion, and therefore a desire to act, is perfectly natural. In my personal view, the expression of that compassion through action, whether within communities or families, is stunted by people genuinely not knowing how to help, despite desperately wanting to. Namaste Care can help close that loop and provide a way to express that compassion gently and lovingly.

Community compassion

In the very early stages of setting up the Namaste Care Project, I was very reluctant to promote it too much before we had a group of trained volunteers in place who could respond to referrals once they started coming in. So my initial attention was on how to attract volunteers to the project. I registered the volunteer opportunity with the local volunteer bureau, and with help from the hospice Communications Officer we did a press release in local newspapers and on social media and I arranged a drop-in session for anyone who might be interested in finding out more.

I need not have worried. The drop-in session was well attended, and my first Namaste Care training session for prospective volunteers filled up quickly. What we have found to be most effective is to invite interested people to attend the day of training before they decide definitely if they want to proceed with volunteering with the project. This way, we have found there is an element of self-selection or de-selection. Participants by the end will all be better informed about how to meet the needs of people with advanced dementia, so in that way, we are slowly strengthening the ability of the community to respond to the growing need. But also it allows people to really check out if they can commit, if they feel confident enough to visit people at home on their own (although I usually support them for the first one or two visits) and whether the project entails what they hoped for.

---

4   Quoted by charterforcompassion.org

By the end of the training, from experience, people are one of three things: enthused and keen to push through with their volunteer application; keen but aware that now might not be the right time for them; or having a rethink about this being the volunteer opportunity for them. I understand that it can feel like a responsibility and it is not for everyone. Some people worry about getting too attached (which you do) or that they will be judged for doing something wrong (which they most certainly won't).

The training covers the following areas, but I know it will evolve and be refined as we continue to learn with the project.

1. Introduction and the meaning of Namaste

2. Dementia awareness

3. Communication – with the person living with dementia and also their carer

4. Progression of dementia and end-of-life issues

5. What is Namaste Care?

6. Group exercise based on case studies

7. Sensory stimulation

8. Learning and practising a simple hand massage technique

Feedback from the training has been really positive. There is always a lovely energy in the room and lots of lively discussion, and even a few tears at some of the moving film clips we use. New friendships between volunteers have grown out of the training too, and even if the potential volunteer does not go on to volunteer, they are able to spread the word about the project and support in other ways, such as fundraising.

From the volunteer application process, safeguards are in place in the form of references, a DBS check and a health check. The volunteers also have monthly access to group supervision, or individual supervision if needed, to share experiences, help one another with ideas and gain support. We have learned a lot together from these supervision sessions, and volunteers have been able to influence and shape how the project has progressed.

Another way to spread the message of Namaste Care is through public speaking, conferences and presentations. I have had to confront my fear of public speaking head on with this one. I have spoken to the Rotary Club, BBC Newcastle Radio, carers groups, at fundraising events, to local community health teams, NHS staff, care agencies, and so on, to share the benefits of Namaste Care, and it is always received with interest. I am not a super-slick public speaker and never will be, but I speak from the heart and with conviction, and as long as you do that, I believe people will listen and care about what you have to say.

As the project progressed, it became very obvious to me that we needed to do some wider dementia awareness work to address the lack of understanding and misconceptions about the condition. We are very lucky to have Ann White MBE as a member of our Namaste Care steering group and now as a Namaste Care volunteer.

Ann received her MBE for her role as chairperson of a highly successful charity committee in Her Majesty's Passport Office, who raised thousands of pounds for local charities. Ann is a Dementia Friends Champion and regularly delivers dementia friends awareness sessions to our hospice staff and volunteers and also the wider community. She is also on the steering group of Dementia Friendly Durham City, helping to make the city a dementia-friendly community. Recently retired, Ann can now devote more time to her roles as this is something very close to her heart. Here are some of Ann's observations:

> Dementia Friends is a global movement that is changing the way people think, act and talk about dementia.
>
> I got involved with Dementia Friends whilst working for Her Majesty's Passport Office. As part of community involvement, they gave me the time to attend the free one-day training session with the Alzheimer's Society in Newcastle in February 2015. My background is in communications and I can be quite critical of training sessions, but this was brilliant. I couldn't help being enthused.
>
> My father was diagnosed with vascular dementia in 2011 and it was a real shock to me and my family. We honestly didn't know where to turn. We were totally ignorant of the disease and like everyone else thought dementia meant just short-term memory loss. I wish I'd known then what I know now, and if I'd attended a Dementia Friends session I would have picked up on Dad's symptoms much earlier instead of simply thinking his falls, confusion and increasing anxiety were down to old age. Sitting in on that first session was like all the pieces of the jigsaw fitting together.
>
> As a Dementia Friends Champion, I'm encouraging people to make a positive difference to people living with dementia in their community. The session covers five key messages helping people to understand that you can

live well with dementia. It also covers the personal impact of dementia and what people can do to help and to reduce the stigma, which unfortunately still exists today. This is because public understanding is very poor and people with dementia often feel, and are, misunderstood, marginalised and isolated. Through these sessions I hope to create a climate of kindness and understanding so that everyone affected by dementia, which includes carers and families of those living with dementia, feels part of society. I know from personal experience how social isolation and loneliness can accelerate dementia. Lack of stimulation and human contact has a massive impact.

Nicola has already mentioned the author Wendy Mitchell. She is an inspiration and has very wise words for both people living with dementia and their families. It's not just the person with the disease who is affected, the diagnosis impacts on everyone in their immediate circle. What disappointed me was that people were scared to visit my father and it was so sad to see his friends drift away, and this left us as a family feeling isolated too. In a way it's like when someone has died. People don't know what to say or how to act and would rather avoid the situation. By raising awareness and understanding we can overcome this, and this in turn will help alleviate the social isolation.

I've also recognised that the older generation are often too proud to accept help and support. This can be down to pride, embarrassment, anger and obviously fear. They have a low level of understanding about dementia and are reluctant to get a diagnosis, and this in turn limits their access to treatment, help and support. They hide away, telling themselves and others that they are fine, but this results in loss of friends, breakdown in relationships and reduced wellbeing. Their scant knowledge is probably from their daily newspaper or watching the TV. The Alzheimer's Society is working hard with the media to change the language they use. Saying a person is 'living with dementia' instead of 'suffering from dementia'. Phrases like 'victim', 'empty shell' and 'living death' are all to create sensationalism to scare people, and so we need to change the way we all talk about dementia.

After all, no one goes from diagnosis to advanced dementia overnight. This can take many years, and with the right medication and support people can live very well with dementia and still enjoy life through travel, hobbies, making new memories and reliving old ones.

Dad eventually had to go into care as we could no longer look after him at home. People thought that this was the end of our worries, but actually all that happened was we swapped one lot of stress for another. The guilt, the fear and the helplessness were immense. Every time we saw news reports of abuse we felt physically sick. After three attempts Dad ended up in a residential home where he was loved and cared for. We still had frustrations, but overall, he was well looked after until his death in 2016.

People were well meaning telling me and my sister to take care of ourselves too. Sometimes I wanted to scream at them and ask them how exactly I was meant to do that. Working full-time in a responsible job, raising a family and caring for Dad was exhausting and at times suffocating. Carers need support too, and kind words are all well and good, but actions speak louder than words. I had immense support in my workplace, and this was invaluable. As a result, I set up a support group in the office for anyone affected by dementia and was heartened to see numerous people gain awareness and give each other support and friendship through the challenging times.

Through the Dementia Friends sessions, I encourage managers to care about the carers in their teams and urge people to visit anyone they know with dementia. Even if it's only for ten minutes, it's a new face and a different conversation and will relieve some of the stress and pressure from the carer.

I love being a Dementia Friends Champion but wanted to do more than just deliver sessions, so a natural progression was to get involved with Dementia Friendly Communities. This has led to being part of the Dementia Friendly Durham City steering group. I work with a cross-section of people from the emergency services, local government, churches, leisure, retail and other organisations, and of course people living with dementia, to help create a culture in which people with dementia and their carers are empowered and supported and feel included in society. This is an exciting venture, and the enthusiasm, passion and collective action within this group is inspiring. We aim to reach out to the many different organisations in the city and encourage them to establish dementia-friendly approaches demonstrating awareness, respect and responsiveness as well as implementing strategies that help people living with dementia. This can be simple things such as providing seating at check-outs in the supermarket or a quiet area in a café, to ensuring signage is dementia-friendly and soft furnishings do not have confusing patterns. Often, it's the simple things that make the biggest difference.

Becoming a Dementia Friend simply means finding out more about how dementia affects a person, and then through this understanding, doing small everyday things that help, and I urge you to find a session in your area by visiting the Alzheimer's Society website. It only takes 45 minutes but can make an immense difference in someone's life. If you cannot find a session then there are videos to watch on the website instead.

Delivering Dementia Friends sessions can be a very humbling experience, and there are often tears but also laughter, and if I've helped only one person through their journey then it's been worthwhile. To date, I've delivered 35 sessions and made nearly 400 dementia friends. I mention my dad in the sessions, and I know he would be proud of my achievement. He is my inspiration, and I will continue to deliver the sessions until everyone in the area is a Dementia Friend or until we have a world free of dementia.

It was Ann who recommended that I ask Ernie Malt, someone living with dementia, to become a member of the Namaste Care steering group, and he has taught me so much about maintaining a positive attitude and driving to keep going with activities for as long as possible. He continues to contribute to his community in so many ways, and as a member of the steering group he ensures that the community focus for the project is always promoted.

As a community, we can support one another better. Greater awareness, sharing resources and knowledge, and a sense of belonging are available to us if we are willing to work towards building compassionate communities.

6

Volunteers with Heart

Barbara Edwards (Namaste volunteer)

In the Namaste Care work at St Cuthbert's Hospice, volunteers play a critical role; indeed, it could not continue without them, given the numbers of referrals being received. The volunteers' visits with the patients at their homes are the central activity of Namaste Care within this project model. In addition, volunteers are the regular point of contact with our patients and their families and are, therefore, liaisons between hospice and family. As a result, the hospice has taken great care to select, train and support the volunteers in their work. This chapter focuses on these elements of our programme and includes some experiences of our current volunteers. The information is based on survey responses and a set of interviews with five volunteers from the programme's first year.

We began by widely advertising the Namaste Care volunteer position in local establishments and on websites of local volunteer organisations. Several volunteers learned about it through their existing connections with St Cuthbert's Hospice, and others saw an article in the local newspaper. The position description included a general statement of the programme, a list of sample activities, and a set of personal characteristics, such as dependability, empathy, ability to maintain confidential information and an interest in advanced dementia.

Applicants were interested in the position for a variety of reasons. Several volunteers had helped family members, neighbours or friends with dementia and had found the time very rewarding. Others had recently retired and were seeking a meaningful volunteer role, and still others had prior positive experiences with St Cuthbert's and were happy to support its work in this specific way. One volunteer was drawn to apply because of the term 'namaste', which she related to her own spiritual journey. As well, most applicants volunteer for other organisations or for St Cuthbert's Hospice in another capacity.

Training and supervision

Potential volunteers were invited to attend a one-day training session to learn more about the programme and the volunteer role. Through presentations and interactive exercises, the training introduced the elements of the Namaste Care Programme, a foundational understanding of advanced dementia as well as good communication skills, a discussion of one's hopes and fears, and the experience of giving and receiving a hand massage, the programme's signature activity. The training day also began the development of the community of volunteers and staff that has been important subsequently for the social and emotional support of each other.

The volunteers found the training day extremely valuable. All volunteers felt that they had deepened their understanding of advanced dementia and improved their communication skills. In particular, they cited the Bookcase Analogy offered in one video clip. Here memory storage is understood as a pair of bookcases representing a set of cognitive memories on one side and a set of emotional memories on the other side. For a person with dementia, books on the top shelves (most recent memories) are the first to fall off, while the oldest memories, those at one's feet, are more stable and long-lasting. The other bookcase contains emotional memories that are stored in a different part of the brain. These are not necessarily affected by dementia. This analogy, offered frequently in presentations by Dementia Friends, helped the volunteers to realise the vitality and importance of the patients' emotional lives even as their cognitive functions are in decline.

The training also included several powerful video clips of sensory stimulation and their profound impact on the patients. In one, an older gentleman named Henry is shown listening to music of his youth. Although he had not spoken or sung for several years, this music brought him to life. His eyes lit up and he began singing along with the music, his face expressing his sheer pleasure. Another similar video clip involves an intense interaction between Naomi Feil, founder of Validation Therapy, and a dementia patient, and the carer's ability to connect with her through, once again, music (see Chapter 14). The carer begins singing a very familiar song, 'Jesus Loves Me', and the patient joins in. The power of the music is clear for these two individuals, but Namaste Care also includes other forms of sensory stimulation that result in similarly powerful moments.

Matching volunteers with patients

When patients are referred to the programme, St Cuthbert's Hospice staff visit the family and conduct a Life Story interview. This information helps the volunteer to know which activities to consider and which ones to avoid (i.e. any with particularly negative associations). Life Stories also help the staff identify the appropriate volunteer by matching areas of interest or backgrounds. An avid gardener will be matched with the patient who loves her plants and flowers. A horse owner will be matched with a patient whose earlier life included all things equestrian. And whenever possible, women are matched with women, and men with men, unless there is a specific request to the contrary. The matching process is considered both on this basis but also on a good deal of intuition, from the point of view of which volunteer will get on well with which person living with dementia and their family.

Visits to the patient's home

During the training day as well as in the interviews, the volunteers shared their fears and concerns about starting this work. Several volunteers said they worried about whether they knew enough (despite the wonderful training) or that they would be inadequate in some respect. One volunteer expressed concern about the intimacy of the touching involved in hand or foot massages. The most common fear expressed was the emotional challenge of developing an attachment to the patient and his or her carers, especially in the face of the patient's decline and eventual death.

Volunteers spend one to two hours per week with their patient. Together they develop a mutually convenient schedule. Some volunteers visit two hours once a fortnight, and others visit for an hour or so each week. For many carers, this is an opportunity for a brief respite from their obligations and a chance to pursue a hobby or read a book. For others, the volunteer's visit is a family affair, and the carer(s) remain in the room to observe their loved one and chat with the volunteer. Each situation is different.

Because dementia is a very individual disease, there is no script or programme of activities that fits all or even most patients. The volunteers spend several visits determining which activities are most appropriate for this particular patient. The volunteers also consider biographical elements they have learned from the patient's Life Story and from conversation with their carers. An animal lover might enjoy looking at pictures of dogs or reading stories about a veterinary practice. A music aficionado might enjoy listening to familiar songs or singing with the volunteer. And many patients enjoy looking at photographs of family members and familiar scenes. So the activities and the rhythm of the visits take time for the volunteer to determine. As the patient's interests and capacities change, the activities the volunteer introduces will change as well.

The volunteers in St Cuthbert's Namaste Care Programme have been imaginative as they select the activities that engage their patient. Based on the information in the Life Story, the capabilities of the patient (e.g. whether they can walk) and other information provided by the carer, the volunteers try out various activities that serve to engage the patient and heighten his/her sensory stimulation. They pay close attention to the patient's responses and preferences. Does he or she like foot massages? Singing hymns? Walking in the garden? Looking at old photographs?

One patient loved baking in earlier years, and so the volunteer engaged her each week in making, baking and, of course, sampling one of her favourite cakes. Another woman used to spend hours in her garden. Though no longer able to garden, she was able to walk with the volunteer in the neighbourhood to appreciate the blooming flowers and plants nearby. Another volunteer guided her patient in knitting projects (you knit a row, I knit a row…), another duo sang beloved Scottish songs, and yet another pair enjoyed working on an adult colouring book. One patient was particularly fond of Gilbert and Sullivan operas and, although bedridden, moved her arms in time to this music when it was played.

For some patients, looking at photographs of loved ones or pets they have owned has been a wonderful and calming activity. For others, viewing pictures has been upsetting, perhaps because they no longer remember who the people in the pictures are, or because it reminds them of their limitations and what they have lost. The volunteer must be sensitive to the patient's emotional response as well as his or her capabilities and interests.

Impact of the work on the volunteers

While the centrepiece of the Namaste Care Programme is the emotional, social and spiritual support of the person with advanced dementia, the impact of the visits on the volunteer is also important. Predictably, the volunteers become attached to the patient (and often to the family members who serve as the carers), and watching the gradual decline and eventual death of the patient is difficult. Volunteers frequently worry about the health of the carer also, especially if that person has underlying health concerns as well.

Despite these challenges, the volunteers find the work very rewarding. There are the small moments, as when the patient reaches out to take the volunteer's hand, or smiles with recognition when the volunteer arrives, or when the carer appreciates the brief but important respite offered by the visit. In general, they feel honoured to be included in this person's life at this important time, and to be trusted by the carers to take them on walks or sing with them or simply develop a friendship.

The Namaste Lead and Admiral Nurse hold monthly supervision meetings with the volunteers to continue training on new topics, share ideas and successes, and offer support for each other. In our programme's first year, for example, two of our patients died, and two others moved into care homes where they no longer receive volunteer visits. The volunteers were grateful to have this caring community with which to share the emotional challenge of these events. As a result of the initial training and these regular meetings, the volunteers feel much more knowledgeable about advanced dementia and much better prepared to offer meaningful support for their patients.

Author's note

Barbara Edwards has been a Namaste Care volunteer since the beginning of the project and has been matched with three different people living with advanced dementia in the course of the project so far. She continues to commit herself to the project despite moving out of the Durham area, and her supportive presence to the project team as well as the people she visits continues to inspire me.

Committing to a Namaste Care relationship requires reliability, compassion and an incredibly kind heart. I have seen volunteers go above and beyond anything I had expected of them, including trips to the library to get books out for the person they visit, baking cakes to take as a treat and many other acts of genuine caring. I am incredibly proud of each and every volunteer.

One touching story recently was when a volunteer helped the person living with dementia that she visits to sign her name on a birthday card for her husband. He was incredibly moved by this as he had never expected to see her write her name again. This simple act speaks of a volunteer who understands the meaning of the many losses a carer can feel and who wanted to help the lady she visits to remind her husband, 'I'm still here.'

I am very aware that we are asking the volunteer not only to connect with the person living with advanced dementia, but also to communicate with and build a relationship with the family. This dual aspect of the role is now covered more thoroughly in training than it was at the beginning of the project.

7

Responding to Referrals – Making Contact, the Initial Visit and Assessment

Obviously, we all know that first impressions count. Making contact with the family following receipt of a referral and explaining the purpose of our project really sets the tone for the rest of our involvement with this family.

We aim to make contact within seven days of receiving a referral and to arrange the initial visit within 15 days. First, I always confirm that they were aware of the referral being made and I ask if it would be convenient to visit them at home so that I can meet the person living with dementia, explain the project to the family, and decide together if we think that it is something that would be helpful.

The most important thing to establish is whether the person's dementia is advanced and that therefore Namaste Care would be appropriate for them. The rate at which dementia symptoms will get worse varies widely and will be different depending on the type of dementia the person has. Alzheimer's, for example, tends to have the slowest rate of progression, but for each person it will also depend on other health conditions, their age, genetics and a host of other factors.

When visiting a person for the first time it is helpful to know what type of dementia they have and when they were diagnosed (this information is requested on the referral form). This will give us a very rough guide to what to expect, and the following information about the different types of dementia gives a brief summary. Above all, getting to know the person is more important, so we also assess the advancement of symptoms from observation and discussion with family.

Types of dementia
Alzheimer's disease

This is the most common form of dementia, which can have a long progression time with several plateaus in symptoms. In late stages, memory loss is very pronounced, with the person often unable to recognise familiar objects, surroundings and people. They may, however, have moments of recognition, which can be encouraged with Namaste Care. The person with late-stage Alzheimer's will most likely be completely dependent on others, with loss of speech, difficulties with eating, drinking and swallowing, weight loss and incontinence. Sometimes there may be irritability, restlessness and aggression, but not always.

Vascular dementia

This can look similar to Alzheimer's but progresses in different ways. There is more of a stepped progression where symptoms are stable and then suddenly worsen. Overall progression (averaging five years) can tend to be more rapid than with Alzheimer's, but the life expectancy in both types will depend on the age the person started with symptoms, as well as other medical conditions and lifestyle.

Dementia with Lewy bodies

Symptoms in dementia with Lewy bodies (related to Parkinson's disease) are far more variable from day to day, and the most predominant issues are related to movement, physical decline, misperceptions, paranoia and the distressing nature of hallucinations. Memory problems may come and go, and some days the person may have insight into their condition which can lead to depression and agitation. People live on average for 6 to 12 years, but this can vary considerably between people.

Not all people with Parkinson's disease will develop dementia, but where dementia symptoms do develop in people living with Parkinson's disease, it is very similar to dementia with Lewy bodies. In both Parkinson's dementia and Lewy body dementia appropriate medication can significantly improve symptoms for a time.

Fronto-temporal dementia

Symptoms of this type of dementia tend to affect either language skills or behaviour, but as it progresses these symptoms begin to blur together and become similar to late-stage Alzheimer's disease. People tend to live on average for between six and eight years with this type of dementia, but again, this can vary.

Rarer forms of dementia

Some people may have a rarer form of dementia that requires a bit of research to understand. We can't be experts in every type of dementia and so we may need information from health professionals and specialists to understand a specific type. For example, progressive supranuclear palsy is a condition characterised by marked muscle stiffness and physical degeneration, a staring facial expression and loss of speech. Other rarer forms of dementia include cortico-basal degeneration, Creutzfeldt-Jakob disease (CJD) and alcohol-related brain damage, amongst many others.

Adapting to the patient and family
Communication needs

It is important to discuss issues related to how the person communicates. This will include checking out whether they need glasses, wear a hearing aid (or are refusing to wear it) and any other relevant factors that we need to be aware of in relation to communication.

Mobility

We also need to understand the person's level of mobility and use of any mobility aids (such as walking frame, hoist or wheelchair). I always make it clear at this point that we would not be expecting volunteers to carry out any moving and handling of the person, and that this would need to be carried out by the family, but that it is useful to know as background information for what the person living with dementia is still able to do physically. This could inform where the person is positioned for visits and any options for moving, for example into the garden.

Continence

Similarly, it is not the role of a volunteer visitor to help with personal care tasks, but it is still useful to know about the person's needs in this area and how they are currently being met. If a person living with dementia wears incontinence pads, they may be more prone to pressure sores, for example, and so we can encourage the family to regularly change the person's seating position.

Memory

I check out what amount of recognition, orientation to time and place, and recall a person has. Often this may be limited to their early life given the late stage of dementia, and so this will inform the volunteer of what era of life to target any reminiscence activities to.

Cognition and behaviour

From discussion with the family, it is usually possible to establish how much the person can follow instructions, what their level of alertness is, and whether they have any unusual behaviours to watch out for. For example, one lady tended to push people away when she became agitated and this could happen suddenly and could take people by surprise. All that was needed was to back off and give her space to calm down and to reassure her.

Sleep

Sleep patterns can provide useful insights into daytime behaviour. Sometimes agitation or tearfulness may actually be linked to poor sleep at night, and lack of daytime stimulation could lead a person to sleep most of the day, thereby sleeping badly at night. We can therefore use this information to support the family to establish a better sleep routine.

Allergies

Given that we may be using massage products, face creams, and so on, we would also check out whether the person has any allergies we need to be aware of, and I always carry out a patch test of products to be used. It is also very important to check out food allergies, considering that we will be encouraging the person to have snacks and drinks.

General health

An overview of the person's other health conditions can be helpful for the volunteer to know. One example we were given was that a lady who was diabetic could develop shaking that did not subside. In this situation, the volunteer was advised to go and alert her husband who would check her blood sugar levels. Other issues we would watch out for would be frequent hospital admissions over the last year, frequent infections, falls and a more frequent need to call the GP. These can be indications that the person is in the final year of life.

History of dependency

We would check out if the person had any history of a dependency on alcohol or drugs, or was a smoker. Even if the person has not had this issue for some time, given the changes in a person's memory, this could influence their current expectations.

Diet and swallowing

It is very important to find out about any dietary requirements so that the volunteer has guidance in this regard. There may be health restrictions we need to be aware of, such as a low-sugar diet for diabetes, or high-calorie requirements for people who are underweight. As dementia progresses, people can develop issues with swallowing and may be now on a pureed diet due to the risk of aspiration (fluid and food being inhaled into the lungs). Frequent chest infections and coughing can be a sign of aspiration, especially when the chest infection is on the lower right lung.

Pain

We would check out whether pain was a known issue for the individual and what makes that pain better or worse. I would also observe the person for any signs of pain, such as grimacing, and ensure the volunteers are aware that they should do the same.

Support being received

I would ask about what care package (if any) the person is receiving from a home care agency, and also whether other professionals such as social workers, community nurses, chiropodists or speech and language therapists are involved. Sometimes it is necessary to get advice from these professionals to offer better support to the family, but I would only do that with permission.

Carer needs

We are well placed to notice where the carer may need additional support, so it usually naturally comes out in the conversation about the carer's own health needs, what support network they have already and whether they are isolated themselves. We can make them aware that they are entitled to a carers' assessment from their local authority if they have not already had one and should be registered at their GP as a carer.

Assessment of risk

Given that we will be sending volunteers into a lone visit situation, we would note any issues related to the safety of the environment, such as smoking, pets, parking difficulties, and so on (see Appendix: Namaste Care Service Referral). If, for example, we became aware that there was a person living in the house with a history of violence, it may not be appropriate to send a volunteer or a lone worker into the house on their own. I also request this information from the person's GP, in case the family fail to disclose issues to me. Consent to share information and to inform the GP of our involvement is discussed at this initial visit. Some risks may be manageable with an agreed plan and with volunteer agreement.

Managing expectations

At this initial visit, I will emphasise that it will be a volunteer who is giving their own time who will visit and that we will need to accommodate the fact that sometimes they will be unavailable due to holidays or sickness. I also discuss the frequency of visits that the family feels is appropriate (usually once weekly or once a fortnight). The boundaries of Namaste Care visits are reinforced when I introduce the volunteer at a later visit, and we all sign the three-way family agreement (see Appendix). I also explain that I am not a nurse, and so at times we may need to draw on the advice available from the Admiral Nurse and that the family can view this as additional support available to them.

By the end of this visit, we should have made a decision together about whether Namaste Care would be helpful, and if so, my next step is to book a date to gather the person's Life Story information.

Matching preferences

If it is established that the referral is appropriate for Namaste Care, I discuss what days, times and other preferences the family may have for matching the volunteer with the person with dementia. For example, often the family will say that it takes the person a while to get up and get sorted in the morning, so late morning or afternoon visits are preferred. We may need to fit around other activities in the week, and the person may have a preference for a male or female volunteer. Whilst I make it clear that it is not always possible to meet all these requests, usually it is possible to meet most of them.

8

Life Stories

If a person lives until the age of 80, they will have over 29,000 accumulated days of a Life Story. That's a lot of life lived. In gathering Life Story information to inform Namaste Care activities, we usually rely on the family to tell us what they know of that person's life, given the memory loss and communication issues that come with advanced dementia. Often, the family weren't there in the childhood of the person with dementia. Maybe their spouse met them in their late teens or early twenties and sons and daughters obviously weren't around to witness the person's early story. So we rely on stories that were told by the person living with dementia over the years to their family and friends about their life.

It would be lovely if we all wrote down our own memories either before or just after a dementia diagnosis. It once happened that I carried out a Life Story session with a family and the lady living with dementia had filled in a memories book bought for her by her daughter. There were some lovely sensory memories in there about watching the flames of an open fire with her friend and trying to see shapes in the flames. Captured moments like this are wonderful snapshots of the things that are important to a person. In this case, the crackling sound of an open fire, the smell of smoke and dimmed lighting might evoke relaxed feelings of cosy nights of friendship and closeness. Whereas, for someone else I explored a Life Story with, the smell of smoke would bring back a traumatic memory of a childhood burning accident, which made every bonfire night stressful for this man living with dementia. These things are important to know, if we possibly can.

So, how do we begin to capture the essence of a life, knowing that we can never hope to know the fine detail?

Every person is a unique and glorious blend of all the physical, emotional, ancestral, spiritual and social aspects that make up who they are. We are all shaped by our genetics, by life events and by our life choices. We are separate individuals, but we are also deeply interconnected and interdependent on others, so it is equally important to know who has been important and influential to the person living with dementia. Tom Kitwood says it this way:

> To have an *identity* is to know who one is, in cognition and feeling. It means having a sense of continuity with the past; and hence a 'narrative', a story to present to others. It also involves creating some kind of consistency across different roles and contexts of a person's life. (Kitwood 1997)

I am very struck by the fact that the person living with advanced dementia becomes unable to do this for themselves in the way that identity is described above, and so they need the people around them to assist them to maintain their identity when they are no longer able to express it easily themselves. This is the main point of Life Story work. To extend the idea that this identity is held by and can be nurtured by others links to Kitwood's discussion of 'personhood': 'It is a standing or status that is bestowed upon one human being, by others, in the context of relationship and social being. It implies recognition, respect and trust' (Kitwood 1997).

Tom Kitwood wrote *Dementia Reconsidered: The Person Comes First* in 1997, and his ideas about the needs of someone living with dementia are very often used to encapsulate the idea of person-centred care. In order to be person-centred, Kitwood describes a cluster of overlapping needs, which he shows in the form of a 'Flower of Need' (see Figure 8.1). Addressing each of these needs will also contribute to fulfilling the others.

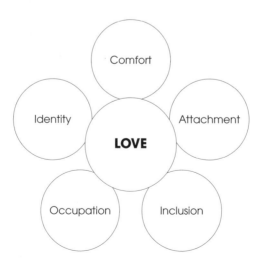

Figure 8.1: Kitwood's 'Flower of Need' (adapted from Kitwood 1997)

- **Comfort** – feeling safe and secure by being close to others and receiving genuine warmth and having pain and discomfort soothed.

- **Attachment** – as social creatures, humans make bonds with others, and it is those attachments that will provide reassurance and a feeling of safety.

- **Inclusion** – we all have a human need for acceptance within a social context and feel a sense of belonging to a group (family, neighbourhood, community, friendship group).

- **Occupation** – when someone has dementia, they still maintain a need to remain useful and needed, otherwise they will feel useless and a burden to those around them. Finding a task the person is able to still do which is meaningful to them based on their Life Story contributes to the sense of inclusion.

- **Identity** – making sure care fits around the person's unique preferences and routines, rather than expecting them to fit into our ideas through the awareness of the life story and the use of empathy.

Holding all of these interconnected needs together is *love*. This is a practical kind of love that values the individual for all that they are and have been. When we love someone we want to spend time with them. When we spend time with them, there is a wordless feeling of warmth between two people that does not require cognitive understanding to appreciate. A person with dementia will retain the ability to feel loved, so we must not be afraid to talk about loving the person with dementia, even in a professional relationship. In my case, I love my Dorothy, the person I visit at home. She looks at me sometimes and I look back, and we have real 'I–thou' moments that I will treasure for as long as I live.

A note of caution

Some people may not enjoy the Life Story process for various reasons. One Life Story I remember completing with a lady who had Parkinson's dementia was covered very efficiently by me, the lady's devoted husband and the volunteer in the presence of the lady herself who was not able verbally to tell us things herself. However, following the Life Story session, she apparently became very down, and when the volunteer visited, she refused to look at photos of the things that we thought were important to her from her past.

What I realised and was mortified about was that the Life Story session had reminded her of all the things she could no longer do and she had insight due to her type of dementia to find this very depressing. I didn't make that mistake again.

The volunteer has found a way to work with her very much in the present moment by sharing hand and foot massages, reading to her and playing music. I now discuss the option of a Life Story with more wariness than before and often the family will know if it is a good idea or not. If it's not, then the family can maybe put together information themselves that would be useful without imposing a Life Story session on a person who might find it difficult. Generally speaking, a Life Story session is enjoyable for everyone involved; however, there will be rare occasions when it is not.

Styles and formats of Life Story

The Alzheimer's Society advocates the use of a simple form called 'This is me', which can be downloaded from their website.[1] They describe it as a 'support tool to enable person-centred care'. It aims to capture important facts about a person's family and cultural background, preferences, key life events and their personality. This form is often given out at diagnosis, but at this point in the dementia journey, it may not be understood for its importance and they tend to remain untouched. This is such a missed opportunity to let health and social care professionals see the person as an individual and better understand their needs.

On a similar but wider theme, a growing movement within the NHS in Scotland is the promotion of 'What matters to you?' conversations.[2] Seeing beyond an anonymous person in a hospital bed is a win-win situation, as it leads to more meaningful interactions for patients and the staff team are able to understand the needs of the person, thus also making their job easier and more fulfilling.

Given there is no definitive way to do a Life Story, the Social Policy and Research Unit at York University (Gridley *et al.* 2015) reviewed literature on the subject and broadly grouped styles of Life Story into the following categories:

- **Chronological** – by focusing on memories and facts, we can try to record a life from birth to now. This could be done in the form of a timeline, for example.

---

1   www.alzheimers.org.uk/get-support/publications-factsheets/this-is-me
2   See www.whatmatterstoyou.scot

- **Narrative** – rather than being purely factual, this includes interpretations and feelings of what has happened and what it has meant to the person.

- **Care focused** – using Life Story work to improve and personalise care, usually in a residential care setting or for the purposes of informing home carers about a person. This will include sections such as how the person likes to be addressed, dietary needs and preferences, medical needs, physical needs (including continence and moving and handling requirements) and a list of visitors/next of kin contacts.

- **Hybrid** – a narrative approach mixed with a care-focused approach to give a very full picture about a person's life history, preferences as well as current care needs. This is the preferred style for our 'My Namaste Care' Life Story format (see Appendix).

This research also identified some good practice principles that are worth sharing when planning to undertake Life Story work.

Learning point 1: It should not be assumed that everyone wants to complete a Life Story, and they should not be forced to do so.

Learning point 2: A person's Life Story is an open, ongoing piece of work and can continue to be added to.

Learning point 3: Life Story work can be sensitive and emotional. Some people may wish to talk things through, some people may not, and this needs to be handled with compassion and understanding.

Learning point 4: A person living with dementia may have a different perspective about their Life Story than others and this view needs to be accepted and valued. If the person is unable to tell us much themselves, as is often the case with advanced dementia, then enlisting the help of someone who knows them well, such as a spouse, is important. It is often necessary to also get the views of siblings or other family members for early life memories.

Learning point 5: It is useful for care staff to create and share their own Life Stories in order to understand the process and how it feels. This would also follow for family members.

Learning point 6: Beginning the process as early as possible will enable the person living with dementia to contribute more to the Life Story, but it is never too late to try.

Learning point 7: A Life Story is only useful if people have access to it and take the time to read and absorb it.

Learning point 8: A Life Story summary may be helpful for busy staff, such as home care workers, but it should not replace having a full, detailed Life Story available.

Being creative

The format we use within the project is a typed form to capture the key information, but there are additional ways that can enhance the process, such as creating photo albums and scrapbooks of notable events through the person's life. These can provide a lovely resource to share with the person living with dementia, creating interaction and interest. Putting together a memory box of items that are significant from across the person's life is also a lovely way to honour who they are. Sports trophies, an old teddy bear, Grandad's pipe – it is entirely personal and unique what can go in a memory box. Some people like to do memory boards that can be displayed, and this is a great visual way to create conversation and interaction with visitors. Personalising a fiddle mitt, blanket or cushion with meaningful items is yet another idea that makes some value from a unique life lived.

Building a Life Story

When building a Life Story, there are simple underpinning themes we are aiming to explore:

- What and who matter to me (past and present)?

- What and who bring me a feeling of comfort and security?

- What might make me feel uneasy?

- What are my practical needs at the moment?

Using a framework that we have called 'My Namaste Care' (which draws on the content of the Alzheimer's Society 'This is me' form mentioned above), under various section headings we set about exploring key aspects of a person's life. The My Namaste Care form (see Appendix) includes suggested areas to cover, but there may be additional important areas you feel need to be covered, so Life Story work should be viewed as a flexible and organic process. Once the form has been completed, I would then give a copy to the family and one to the volunteer (with permission), keep a copy on file, and encourage the family to make the Life Story available to home carers or to health care staff should the person require a hospital admission.

Sporting memories

If the person living with dementia was involved with sport, this can provide a wealth of rich reminiscence material to explore. Think about the tactile nature of sports equipment such as the old laced footballs or a cricket ball. Trophies, photographs and social contacts with old team members are all really useful information to gather. At St Cuthbert's Hospice, we run a Sporting Memories group and there is information and support with regard to information, training and resources via the Sporting Memories Foundation Network.[3]

Sport really can be a means to tackle isolation, depression and feelings of hopelessness. Remembering achievements and celebrating them can really serve to lift a person living with dementia. The same disclaimer, however, applies to people who would feel this to be a reminder of what they have lost, as previously discussed.

By way of concluding this chapter on Life Story work, I want to quote the research team at York University:

> Everybody has a life story. These are rich and varied and can be used to communicate who we are to the people around us. People with dementia sometimes need help to communicate their histories and identities, and it has been suggested that life story work could present a way for them to do this more easily. (Gridley *et al.* 2015)

I would simply say, give it a try. A family's history is a valuable shared legacy that can help the younger generations make sense of events, understand the person with dementia and value them for the unique person they are.

---

3   www.sportingmemoriesnetwork.com

9

Psychological Needs of People with Advanced Dementia

Early in the Namaste Care Project, I visited a couple to carry out a Life Story, which was heavily reliant on the husband telling me about his wife's life, given how advanced her dementia had become. This lady tended to sleep a lot of the time and did not speak very often, but when she did, it was usually unclear what she was trying to say verbally (although I noticed she was conveying a lot non-verbally). Her husband told me, however, that if she burped when he was helping her with her meals, she would very clearly say, 'Oh, do excuse me.' She had always been a very quiet, polite and well-mannered lady, and it was obvious that this was still important to her and the habitual verbal response to burping was still available to her.

This got me thinking about the importance of knowing, really knowing, who each person is and what matters to them. What has made them who they are, and how can we honour their beliefs when we spend Namaste time with them? As a qualified psychotherapist, I understand the important legacy of our childhood influences in making us who we are, and so using the model of Transactional Analysis, we can begin to explore this in more depth.

Transactional Analysis

Transactional Analysis is a theory of personality that was developed by psychiatrist Eric Berne (1910–1970), and it gives us a way to understand how people are structured psychologically and how this influences behaviour. I was intrigued to learn how dementia may affect the model of personality

I was taught in my psychotherapy training. Berne describes three basic parts of our personality, which are formed in early life (before the age of seven). He called these 'ego states' (see Figure 9.1).

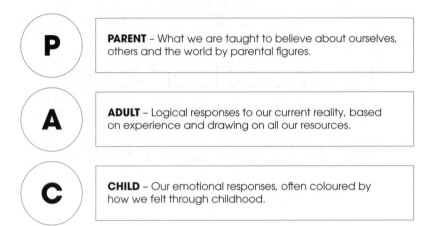

P

PARENT – What we are taught to believe about ourselves, others and the world by parental figures.

A

ADULT – Logical responses to our current reality, based on experience and drawing on all our resources.

C

CHILD – Our emotional responses, often coloured by how we felt through childhood.

Figure 9.1: The structure of ego states (adapted from Berne 1961)

For a thorough explanation of the fully developed theories of Transactional Analysis, see Stewart and Joines (2003).

Honouring the 'Parent'

Imagine all the subtle and not so subtle ways our parents, grandparents, teachers and other important people in our early life moulded us and influenced us. Even if that led to our rebelling and doing the opposite of those things, that decision itself is still in response to this early teaching. Here are some simple examples:

'You **should** keep your feelings to yourself.' (*Be strong.*)

'You **should** do everything perfectly.' (*Be perfect.*)

'You **shouldn't** keep other people waiting.' (*Hurry up.*)

'You **should** put other people's needs before your own.' (*Please others.*)

'You **should** always work hard and do your best.' (*Try hard.*)

The list is unique to each person and would have been reinforced by verbal and non-verbal messages (watch out for 'that disapproving look' from mother!). The messages were not necessarily right (such as 'You should always look after others before yourself'), but they can become ingrained and accepted as if they were true. This is how prejudices such as racism and sexism are passed down through families.

It became clear to me that as we get to know someone through the project, we need to get a sense of the type of person they are and, in a non-judgemental way, respect their beliefs, even if they are contrary to our own.

As a personal example, my grandad was racist. My wonderful grandmother quietly counteracted his messages to me by buying me a black doll to play with and by frowning and shaking her head subtly whenever he said something racist. However, for his own reasons he believed what he believed, and so it would have been counter-productive for both sides to have matched him with a volunteer from a Black, Asian or Middle Eastern ethnicity, uncomfortable as this is to acknowledge.

Another example was when I was asking a family about permission to take photographs. The husband told me that his wife who was living with dementia had always been a very modest, private person who didn't like her photograph taken, but that she would be unable to object now, so it was fine. I gently pointed out that it would be better for us to respect her preferences and to forget the photographs. They were, after all, for the benefit of the project and not for her.

See the Appendix for a short but revealing questionnaire called 'Who Am I?' that can get at some of these messages from childhood which continue to influence us. Ideally, this would be most beneficial to be completed by asking the person with dementia as early as possible in their dementia journey, otherwise the answers will rely on what the person has told their family about their childhood.

Supporting the 'Adult'

Our 'Adult' ego state is the rational, clear-thinking, 'seeing the whole picture' part of us, and is based on what we have learned from experience. This seems to me to be the part of a person most profoundly affected by dementia. Decision-making, planning, motivation, independence and ability to manage tasks give way to confusion, difficulty in sequencing a task, loss of confidence and reliance on others.

There are some things that are worth a try to help with memory, such as labelling things, creating a routine, minimising distractions, helping the person feel oriented to times of day and establishing gentle rhythm to each day, but what works will be very individual to each person.

We have a very inspiring man who is living with dementia on our steering group. His name is Ernie Malt and he is a true force of nature, determined to do as much as he can, for as long as he can. When I first met Ernie, he was working on building a sensory garden in the grounds of his local church. He was still driving at the time and he attended our Namaste training so that he could spread the approach into his local care homes. However, I have always been acutely aware of the bravery of this man to be involved in supporting my project as a steering group member, as what I was asking him to consider was his own future.

Listening to him talk about his fears for the future helped me to clarify in my mind what is essentially a fear of the loss of 'Adult' ego state functioning. Ernie worries about the time when he is no longer in control. He worries that he will have needs that he will be unable to communicate and he will be totally reliant on others to care for him. This therefore reinforced to me the need to give people with advanced dementia as much choice and control as possible, and to respond to their non-verbal ways of telling us what they want and need, if they are unable to verbally tell us. For example, I once took a yogurt to my Dorothy as a treat when I visited and her crinkled facial expression told me very quickly she didn't like it. She didn't have to say! I stuck to her favourite chocolate mousses after that.

One of the common things I see when I visit people at home is the family carer trying to prompt the person living with dementia to remember something. 'Of course you remember who that is' I often hear as we look through old photographs or talk about memories from the past. This is a complicated and emotional issue for the family member. They want to try to jog the person's memory, to prove it's still in there somewhere, to keep them stimulated and prevent the memory loss. But imagine how the person living with dementia feels to be told 'That's your son Keith'. I would imagine that this is one of the worst fears for people living with dementia, to forget those closest to them. So, I would advise taking the pressure off expecting things from the person as being much more helpful. Reducing distractions, not bombarding them with questions, simplifying life as much as possible, will help the person to feel less at odds with their current situation.

I think that, for all concerned, moving from thinking as the main functioning strategy, to one of feeling and emotion, requires acceptance and understanding, that this is just how it is. Once this is accepted, the emphasis can be on creating an environment that will generate positive, peaceful feelings, rather than expecting the person living with dementia to be able to continue to perform tasks, recall events, listen to reasoning, and so on.

This often requires a switching of roles within relationships and families, which can be a challenge when, for example, the person who now has dementia has always sorted out the finances.

Loving the 'Child'

In most childhoods, there will be the things that helped us to feel relaxed, safe and loved, and other things that maybe made us feel anxious, sad or angry. These things reside within our 'Child' ego state and can operate like an elastic band, rebounding us back to those old feelings when something happens in the present that is similar to and triggers that particular feeling. Think of the feeling you get when you think of a much-loved parent or grandparent who made you feel loved, compared to the feeling of the memory of a scary neighbour who wouldn't give you your ball back.

So maybe think about dementia this way. Imagine how you felt on your first day at school. You wake up and you really don't know what to expect. You are taken to a place that you don't know, it is unfamiliar and you are asked to do new things, not knowing what is expected of you. The faces around you are strangers and you feel very isolated. The thing that over time reduces your anxiety is familiarity, routine, and knowing how to act and what to do. But most of all, the presence of a steady, reliable, calm and soothing caregiver of some kind (parent, grandparent, childminder, teacher, etc.) who is guiding you will help you feel that maybe school isn't so scary after all.

Translating this into supporting someone living with dementia, as Joyce Simard reinforces time and again, we just need to create a gentle routine, and love them.

The Alzheimer's Society, as part of their Dementia Friends training, has an excellent way to explain this concept, which bears repetition (Barbara Edwards mentions it in Chapter 6). The Bookcase Analogy can be viewed on their website and on YouTube, and is well worth a watch as it makes understandable why a loving approach will work. It goes like this:

> *Each of us has a part of the brain called the hippocampus, which stores facts, essentially like a narrative of memories from our lives. So imagine that beside us we have a bookcase, which is as tall as we are, and which stores all these facts and memories. The only thing is, this bookcase is a fairly flimsy, flatpack variety, and when dementia hits it, this bookcase will start to rock. Books will start to fall from the shelves, starting from the top, which are our most recent memories, and moving down through the years until maybe all that remains*

are some memories from our teens or childhood. This is why someone with dementia may not be able to remember what they ate for lunch, but could tell you what meal their mother made them when they were ill, or the colour of the tablecloth on Granny's dining table.

However, we do have another storage system, called the amygdala, which stores our emotions and feelings in response to our experiences. Now imagine the amygdala as a strong, solid oak bookcase on the other side of us. This bookcase is not so affected by dementia, and doesn't rock very much at all.

So, if you were to visit the person living with dementia, and have a blazing argument, maybe born out of frustration or worry, and you storm out leaving them crying, you might reassure yourself that they won't remember the argument. The truth is they probably won't. But the next time they see you, they will remember the feeling, and may well become distressed. Conversely, if you visit and you pamper them, maybe take them out to sit in the spring sunshine in the garden amongst the trees or have a lovely ride out in the car, then even though they might not remember the details of your visit, they will remember the warm, loved, cared-for feelings that they will associate with you. (Summarised in my own words.)

Put simply, feeling loved and cared for will evoke a sense of safety, of being valued and feeling peace. I am sure all family members and carers would want this for the person they are caring for, it's just that the stress of caring gets in the way a lot of the time. The needs of the carer will be considered in more detail in Chapter 11.

Behaviour changes

An issue which families can find distressing is when the person living with dementia begins to behave in ways that they haven't previously in life. This provides an extra challenge to 'honouring the spirit within'. For some people, symptoms of dementia may include disinhibition, and so the person may begin to display socially inappropriate behaviour where they never did before. This can include shouting out and swearing, brutal honesty, physical and verbal aggression, sexually inappropriate behaviour, undressing in public, and so on. Although much worried about, it is a less common problem than the often-held perception of dementia. More often than not, by the time symptoms are advanced the person is more passive and apathetic. However, if these behaviour changes are present, we need to consider how to support the person with them as they can potentially put incredible strain on relationships within families.

Previously termed 'challenging behaviour', there is growing understanding within care that this behaviour can indicate an unmet need or is a symptom of the dementia that the person is unable to control. Encouraging families to see the behaviour as the dementia, not the person, can be helpful. Also, trying to work out what the unmet need that drives the behaviour might be is a useful approach. For example, aggression or constant tearfulness may indicate pain, a urine infection, boredom or fear. It's not always possible to identify a cause, but when we do it is often then possible to address it.

Thinking again about the ego states previously described, if a person living with dementia was swearing or being sexually inappropriate, for example, it is possible to speak to them from our own 'Parent' ego state to inform them that this is not okay by speaking to their 'Child' ego state. It is perfectly okay to calmly and firmly tell someone that this is not the way to behave in the way a kindly parent or grandparent may have done (see Figure 9.2).

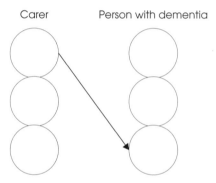

Figure 9.2: Nurturing the 'Parent' ego state speaking directly to the 'Child' ego state

Distraction is also a good way to address some of this behaviour, and so studies into Namaste Care have consistently shown a reduction in aggression and agitation amongst residents in care homes by providing a supportive and meaningful activity. Given the concern about this aspect of dementia, however, I have asked Julie Young to give us more detail about how to support a person with behaviour changes in the next chapter.

The core skill for someone supporting a person living with dementia is therefore empathy. It is vital to have the ability to imagine what life must be like living with memory loss and confusion, not recognising your surroundings or those people around you. Empathy builds the patience required to calmly answer the same question 20 times a day and to know that this behaviour is not the total sum of this person, merely an expression of their illness.

10

The Needs-Led Model of Dementia Care

Julie Young (Advanced Nurse Practitioner, Northumberland, Tyne and Wear NHS Trust)

Dementia is a progressive disease, and the person's ability to reason, make decisions and communicate can deteriorate as their dementia progresses. The person's skills with regard to daily living activities may also deteriorate, and the person may experience a different reality due to the loss of memories and a lack of recognition of what is familiar to them. This may lead to the person with dementia attempting to meet their physical and emotional needs without the ability to articulate what they are doing. This can then result in behaviours which are deemed challenging to carers, such as aggression, shouting and swearing, and increased restlessness, leading to both the person with dementia and their carer becoming distressed.

Historically, the culture of dementia care, known as traditional dementia care, had been dominated by the 'biomedical approach' (Rolfe 1996), which considers dementia in terms of brain pathology. Care was focused on dementia as a 'disease', so interventions were grounded in the 'standard neurogenic disease paradigm' (Moniz-Cook, Stokes and Agar 2003) with a dominant use of medication. Traditional dementia care (Chenoweth et al. 2009) focused on carrying out task-oriented physical care based on the activities of daily living (i.e. the monitoring of diet and the delivery of personal care). The influence of psychosocial and environmental factors in the causation and maintenance of behaviours that were deemed challenging was not considered relevant, and the subjective experience of living with dementia went unrecognised. It was a commonly held view that the presentation of challenging behaviour in individuals with dementia was an inevitable consequence of the disease process.

This approach to care, where the management of behaviour, rather than understanding the reasons for it happening, was the primary focus of attention, resulted in neglect of the person's psychosocial and emotional needs (Kitwood 1997). It did not address the complexity of dementia or the need for an integrated care approach to maintain the wellbeing of a person with dementia (Chenoweth *et al.* 2009; Kitwood 1997).

The needs-led perspective offers an alternative framework to traditional care for understanding the person with dementia and takes account of the 'whole' person. The merits of a needs-led approach to dementia care are supported by the NICE guidelines (NICE 2006, updated in 2018),which endorse the rationale for developing a person-centred approach to dementia care. This is considered best practice for people with dementia (Kitwood 1997).

A needs-led perspective is underpinned by the philosophy that the function of behaviours that challenge can be seen as a communication of a need that is not being met (Jackman and Young 2013). Cohen-Mansfield (2001) suggested that behaviours that challenge can be seen as unmet need, with three possible ways in which unmet need translates into behaviour – the function of the behaviour being:

- an attempt by the person to meet a need; for example, a person who feels hungry may take food from another person's plate in a care home setting

- an attempt by a person with dementia to communicate to others; for example, shouting for help, pressing a buzzer or calling for the police

- a response to their attempt to meet the need being thwarted; for example, the person with dementia becomes aggressive when someone tries to stop them leaving a building.

Considering needs rather than problems reflects a person-centred approach, where interventions are aimed at wellbeing rather than at preventing problems; that is, making the behaviour unnecessary rather than trying to stop behaviour that is already happening (Jackman and Young 2013). A needs-led approach enables care to be tailored to meet psychosocial as well as physical needs. It recognises that physical, psychosocial and emotional needs can result in behaviours that are an attempt by the person to meet these needs; however, due to their being unable to clearly articulate what they are doing, it can result in behaviours that others can find challenging and difficult to understand. This perspective allows a raft of interventions to be considered that empower those who care for people with dementia to try to identify and address the unmet need. When interventions are put in place that meet the need of the person, they can reduce the behaviour and improve wellbeing. The traditional care approach, which simply accepted behaviour as a symptom of the dementia, restricted and limited options to ignoring the behaviour or trying to stop the behaviour often through medication.

The Newcastle Model (James and Stephenson 2007) is a needs-led biopsychosocial model that provides both a framework and a process to work with. It has been developed by bringing together a variety of psychological models (Beck 1976; Cohen-Mansfield 2000; Kitwood 1997). The framework (see Figure 10.1) contains contextual information about the person with dementia and specific details of the behaviour (James and Stephenson 2007).

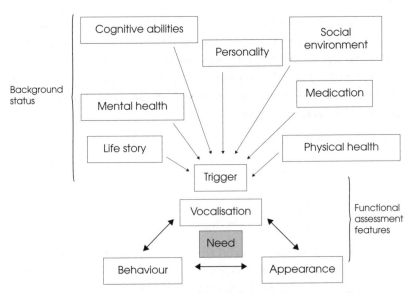

Figure 10.1: The Newcastle Model. A framework for understanding challenging behaviour (James and Stephenson 2007)

It is important to understand clearly what the person with dementia is doing and saying at the time of the behaviour, as well as how they look, in order to be able to assess the person's thoughts and feelings, which then helps us understand the function of this behaviour. This triad is linked to the triggers as to when this behaviour is most likely to occur (see Figure 10.2).

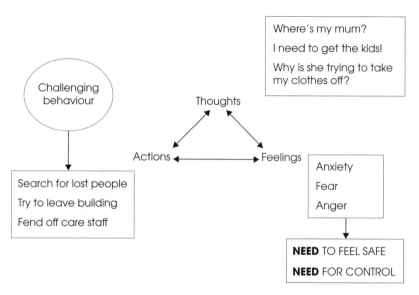

Figure 10.2: Cognitive behaviour maintenance cycle –
The Newcastle Model (James et al. 2006)

The process consists of assessment and formulation of the person's needs. This is most beneficial when done in an information-sharing session with carers of the person with dementia and families to enable a better understanding of the behaviour of the person and their needs. This enables interventions to be developed that can meet these needs. Our challenge when working with people with more advanced dementia is to understand the message and engage with the need not being met:

- What is the person trying to tell us?

- Why in this way?

- What needs are not being met?

- How can we meet this person's needs?

The Newcastle Model (James and Stephenson 2007) guides a structured assessment that can be informed by Maslow's Hierarchy of Needs (Maslow 1943). Maslow believed that people were always seeking to fulfil their potential and that they experience anxiety and discomfort when their needs are not met. It is often presented as a pyramid, with physical needs forming the base, moving up to the ultimate fulfilment of self-actualisation. Maslow believed that only when one level was satisfied could the person move to the next level (see Figure 10.3).

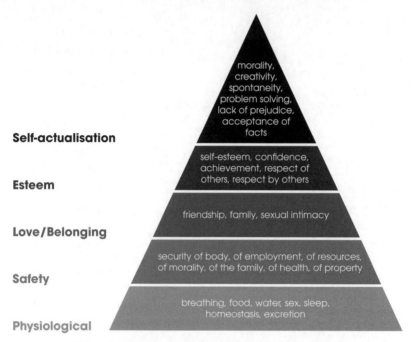

Figure 10.3: Maslow's Hierarchy of Needs (Maslow 1943)

With this structure in mind, physiological needs, which include food, drink and warmth, will take precedence over the need for occupation if they are not met. Likewise, unresolved pain can lead to problems such as depression and hitting out during care interventions. The second level of Maslow's hierarchy is the need for safety. Safety needs may include the physical need for safety in a secure environment, but can also mean psychological safety, where the person feels safe in a consistent familiar and stable environment. The third level is belonging, where people with dementia may follow carers and staff trying to seek out people they are familiar with in an attempt to meet this need, which can also lead to withdrawal from others. The next level is for status and self-esteem, something on which dementia can have a devastating effect. For example, someone can become very distressed when they cannot recall being visited by family and can refuse to accept explanations, making them feel isolated and abandoned, with little self-worth. It is worth bearing in mind that some argue that this structure suggested by Maslow (1943) is too rigid and simplistic as we do not all follow such a linear hierarchy with our psychological needs (Naumof 2017), but it is nevertheless a helpful way to consider needs.

Interventions

As a result of identifying a person's needs, interventions can be devised that are person-centred. Non-pharmacological interventions are recommended as best practice (NICE guidelines), and only when these are not successful should pharmacology (medication) be considered. Examples of identified needs and interventions:

CASE STUDY – MR JONES

Mr Jones would try to leave his home at three o'clock in the afternoon believing he had to take the dog for a walk, a dog they no longer had. *Identified needs*: Purpose and occupation. *Interventions*: He was assisted to go for a walk at this time and would engage with his wife following this by helping to set the table and doing some dishes.

CASE STUDY – MRS SMITH

Mrs Smith would become extremely distraught when staff would try and assist with personal care. *Identified needs*: Pain relief, to feel safe and have her dignity maintained. *Interventions*: Pain relief was offered one hour before assistance to get out of bed, as she suffered from arthritis in her shoulders, making movement uncomfortable. Only female carers assisted her and only those who had developed a rapport with her and whom she was familiar with, and who knew about her Life Story and personality, so they had topics they could discuss which were specific to her. Whilst changing or bathing she would keep a towel around her to maintain her dignity.

When considering needs and advanced dementia it has become helpful to consider the overall need for comfort, which can be addressed using the Newcastle Model and the formulation process and also taking into consideration Maslow's Hierarchy of Needs.

A needs-led, person-centred approach lends itself well to the holistic approach adopted in palliative care as it looks at the whole person. Asking the question 'What gives that person comfort?' enables the care delivery to be tailored to someone's physical, psychosocial and spiritual wellbeing at the end of their life (Young, Gilbertson and Reid 2017), with evidence showing that a more personal approach to comfort has improved patient care, particularly with improved communication with families and caregivers (Arcand *et al.* 2009). Reframing the person with dementia's distress as a need for comfort can enable family and care staff to explore what this means for the person and consider interventions to meet this need.

The collaborative approach between dementia care and palliative care supports those working in dementia care to incorporate the principles of palliative care into their practice (Gibson *et al.* 2009). There is an emphasis on the need for the person with dementia and their carers to receive co-ordinated, compassionate and person-centred care, including access to palliative care (Department of Health 2009, 2015; NHS England 2014).

Below is a case study outlining how a care plan was developed around the need for comfort supported by the Newcastle Model and Maslow's Hierarchy of Needs. The details have been changed to protect the identity of the individual.

CASE STUDY – JACK

Jack was living in a care home and was living with advanced Alzheimer's disease. He had severe dysphasia, communicating through shouting and screaming frequently during the day and night. This impacted on other residents in the home, which the care home staff and family found very distressing. He had severely reduced oral intake, with an impaired swallowing reflex and postural difficulties, which also impacted on his ability to eat and drink. Jack had impaired balance and was no longer able to walk, spending time either in his bed or his chair.

His GP had had a discussion with the family that Jack was potentially approaching the end of his life, and he had reviewed Jack's pain relief. The GP had sought advice from the consultant psychiatrist with regard to further advice about medication for Jack's agitation and distress, which continued despite the pain relief. Due to his ongoing distress, it was felt appropriate to consider a needs-led assessment for further support and the development of non-pharmacological interventions.

Information-sharing session

A session was carried out in the residential home with members of staff and hospice staff. Information was shared regarding Jack's Life Story, personality, social environment, mental health, physical health, cognitive abilities and medication.

During the session we discussed the reasons why Jack was shouting out, what he said, what he looked like at this time and how he behaved. We looked at triggers to this distress, which included certain staff interventions, certain times of day, frustration, despair, perseveration, pain, constipation and possible infection and delirium. Within the session, the word 'comfort' was mentioned several times.

To explore the concept of comfort further, the 'daisy loop' (Pearce 1999) was used to consider what people understood by the term comfort. We explored the different perceptions of comfort held by those at the session and what the perceptions of other professionals who were not present might be. We discussed how Jack might perceive comfort, and the staff from the hospice asked the question 'How did that person previously seek comfort and what did comfort mean to the person?' This exercise highlighted the different perceptions of comfort and what it could mean to Jack, ranging from being infection-free, taking medication and listening to music (see Figure 10.4).

The framework of the Newcastle Model looked at the following areas in relation to comfort: Life Story, personality, physical health, mental health, cognitive ability, medication and social environment. With this information we considered what interventions might be appropriate for the Comfort Care Plan. Maslow's Hierarchy of Needs was used as a guide to ensure that physical and emotional health needs were met.

The Comfort Care Plan detailed the specific interventions that staff could offer Jack, and some of the interventions are given in Table 10.1. The care plan also outlined the support required from other relevant professionals, including the GP, Community Mental Health Team, physiotherapist, occupational therapist and hospice staff.

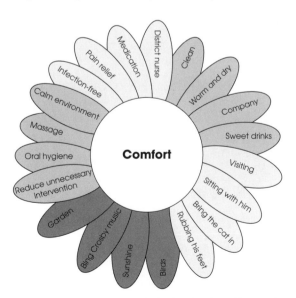

Figure 10.4: Jack's 'daisy loop' acknowledged as developed by Northumberland Tyne and Wear NHS Foundation Trust (adapted from Pearce 1999)

Table 10.1: Jack's Comfort Care Plan

Social environment comfort	Personality/Life Story comfort
• Being outside in the sun – staff would wrap Jack up and take him in the garden in the wheelchair. • See the sun – so his bed was moved to the window. • Hear the birds – when the window was open, he could hear the birds with a birdfeeder put outside his window. • Photographs of his family were put on the wall so he could see them from his bed and staff could talk about them. • He liked a small bedside light on at night or at dusk. • Staff would sit with Jack other than when carrying out physical health tasks. • He liked a red fleecy blanket around his shoulders.	• Family visits – home supporting visits providing meals and drinks for family. • Jack loved Bing Crosby songs – staff and family ensure that this is provided for him. • He has always felt the cold and liked to wear socks in bed – staff and family ensure this is followed. • He likes his back rubbed and feet rubbed. • His family would bring his cat in to sit on his knee to be with him.

A needs-led model therefore requires dialogue between those around a person and a bit of detective work, but it can make a huge difference to the quality of life of someone living with advanced dementia.

11

Carer Needs

Throughout 2017 to 2018 it became increasingly obvious that my dad, now in his late eighties, was developing symptoms of dementia. As is so often the case, he steadfastly refused to discuss this with the GP, finding the idea of possibly having dementia embarrassing and scary. He finally saw a GP in December 2018 and so began the diagnosis process and the involvement of services, the whirl of appointments and professionals, the 'overwhelm' of information. Following his six-week hospital admission in January 2019 with delirium, I learnt firsthand the true depth of stress carers can experience.

What makes us acquire this label of 'carer'? The people I meet who are caring for someone living with advanced dementia are husbands, wives, sons, daughters, grandsons, granddaughters. They are caring for the person because they love them and feel it is their job. Few really identify with 'carer' as a title of what they do. Often, despite being entitled to a carer assessment via social services to support them in their caring role, many have not accepted this offer, or even know about it. They do the best they can, for as long as they can, and then often a crisis happens, which is when 'services' swoop in and it can all seem very confusing and overwhelming with the number of different agencies involved. Carers become keeper of the appointment calendar, steward of daily medication, dietician, chef, housekeeper, head gardener, health care assistant, advocate, and so much more. This carrying of the responsibility can feel very lonely, stressful and draining. As the person living with dementia becomes more socially isolated because they find it difficult to leave the house, then so does the carer, if they can't leave the person unattended.

By the time we have reached the advanced dementia stage, carers have been on a long and stressful dementia journey, which could have included their loved one wandering, unwise financial decisions, lost paperwork, frequent falls and health emergencies, amongst many other possible scenarios. Interestingly, what carers often tell me is that they find this stage of dementia a bit easier, especially if the person is no longer able to walk. Although the personal care tasks, meal making and so on remain, they know that once the person is seated then they are relatively safe, and this reduces the need for such a high level of constant vigilance at least. However, this does also mean that they are so physically tired by the other tasks they have carried out, they have very little energy left for providing stimulating activities and for the idea of Namaste Care. I think this in part accounts for their willingness for others to try out this approach with their loved one, and their reluctance to do it themselves. It could also be that this is not how they view their relationship with the loved one. My hope would be if a carer looks after themselves, then some Namaste Care can actually be mutually beneficial for both the carer and the person they are caring for.

Overwhelmingly, carers need reassurance that they are doing the right things. Most have never had any experience of carrying out personal care tasks and have to learn quickly how to meet the needs of the person they are caring for. I have helped people with personal care many times in my working life, but that did not prepare me for having to help my proud and fiercely private dad to the toilet. But the reality is that the carer knows that person better than anyone else, and if that person can no longer easily express their needs, then the carer becomes their voice.

It is a well-known saying that you cannot pour from an empty cup. Carers must be supported to see that it is not selfish to consider their own needs, as this enables them to stay well and continue to care for as long as possible. So based on our experience with Namaste visits and getting to know carers, I can make some suggestions about the kinds of things that can support carers, but acknowledge that everyone is different, and what works for one person may not suit another.

Maintaining good physical and mental health

It's surprising how many carers neglect their own wellbeing because they are so focused on the person they care for. Often the frequency of appointments for the person they care for means that it can feel an added burden to attend appointments for themselves as well. A key thing as a carer is to ensure you register with the GP as being a carer, and this will alert the GP to monitor and support how you are doing, given how important it is for you to stay well. Personal care tasks can be heavy on joints, and sore backs are very common as you may never have been taught good moving and handling techniques. Nipping any niggles like this in the bud by asking the GP for a referral to a physiotherapist is a wise move, and then doing any exercises they suggest regularly will help you maintain good physical wellbeing.

Similarly, it is easy to put off when you are busy with caring for others, but getting ailments of any sort checked out promptly will be an investment in yourself and will consequently benefit the person you care for too. One issue I hear about this is that it can be tricky to leave the house when you are caring for someone with advanced dementia. Do you leave them for a short while, take them with you (which can be logistically difficult) or get someone to sit with them? Again, no one else can tell you the best way to organise this, but I would say if it is possible to get someone to sit with the person with dementia to enable you to attend an appointment, this will allow you to focus on yourself for this short time and you are more likely to have most productive use of the time.

The stressful nature of caring can inevitably lead to anxiety, insomnia, depression and other kinds of mental health conditions. There will be mental health services in your area who can offer counselling support and a listening ear when you need to share how you feel. Your GP should be able to give you information about this. Often it is easier to tell a stranger how you really feel, especially if you are struggling, whereas people often don't want to worry family and friends by offloading all their thoughts and feelings. Normalising any feelings you do have is so important to avoid the guilt that seems to go with caring. It is normal to feel angry, sad, frustrated and hopeless. A couple look forward to a retirement where they spend time together doing the things they always planned, not having to live with a life-limiting condition. A son or daughter looks forward to their parents witnessing their life events – maybe a marriage, house move, children, career – not to watching a parent decline physically and cognitively. None of us are prepared, and so the sense of unfairness and 'if only' can be very real and painful.

Most people are aware of the signs of stress and burnout, but fewer people have heard of another consequence of caring, which is compassion fatigue. Compassion fatigue develops over time and is a result of a strain being put on our need to empathise with the person being cared for. It is harder to spot in ourselves, but a summary of the types of symptoms to look out for are set out in Table 11.1.

Table 11.1: Negative consequences of caring

Stress	'The engine is revving!'	• Headaches • Upset stomach • Tight chest, rapid heart • Muscle tension • Difficulty relaxing • Speaking quickly
Burnout	'There's nothing left in the tank!'	• Chronic fatigue • Forgetfulness • Insomnia • Loss of appetite (or comfort eating) • Dizziness • Anxiety, depression • Isolation
Compassion fatigue	'My caring is stretched beyond its limit and I'm not taking care of myself!'	• Feeling overwhelmed • Feelings of hopelessness • Feeling inadequate • Lack of empathy • Disengaged, uninterested • 'What's the point?' • Being over-involved/worrying about the problems of others

The remedy for all of these issues is giving yourself permission to take regular breaks and to continue to build into the week the things that you enjoy.

It's also important to acknowledge though that it is not all negative. Often carers feel a strong sense of purpose and enjoy being needed, even enjoy learning new things about caring that they hadn't known before. By the end of their caring journey, carers have acquired a lot of knowledge and often feel a sense of achievement. They may feel able to enjoy using their strengths in the caring role, such as their caring nature, their organisational skills or their communication skills. Sons and daughters have told me that dementia has meant them spending more time with a parent and doing nice things with them than they might otherwise have done if they were well. Writing down at the end of each day something that you have enjoyed or are grateful for can help you notice the positive side of caring too.

Being mindful

Learning mindfulness techniques can be a very useful way to manage the stress of a caring role. Jon Kabat-Zinn (1996) defines mindfulness as 'paying attention, in a particular way, on purpose, in the present moment, and non-judgementally'.

Mindfulness is a way of tuning in to our experience from moment to moment. By observing our thoughts, physical sensations and emotions, we can learn to listen to the information they give us to make wiser choices, rather than reacting out of habit or pre-learned negative beliefs. By living in the present moment, we do not dwell in the past or worry about the future, but we live in all that is real right now.

We spend so much time feeling anxious about 'what if' and imagined future scenarios that may never happen, or dwelling and ruminating on the past and wishing it was different, that we miss the here and now, which could be a very special shared moment with your loved one with dementia, a beautiful sunrise, birdsong or whatever other beautiful moment that life presents us with, and we brush over, focusing instead on the negatives. If 20 things happen in a day, some of them positive, some neutral and one or two negative, what is it we focus on and think about? Pausing instead and allowing the positive moments to really absorb and seep in to our very being will redress this negativity bias and lift our mood.

An extremely useful mindfulness exercise, which only takes a few minutes and should be practised three times a day (think of it like taking your medicine), is the 'Three Step Breathing Space'. Used regularly over time, this technique will increase resilience to stress and allow you to learn a way to deal with stressful situations. (NB. Do not use this technique if you are experiencing very severe anxiety, depression or thoughts of suicide.)

Three Step Breathing Space

Take a **pause** from what you are doing and change your posture in some way, ideally sitting up straight in a chair with feet planted on the floor and shoulders relaxed.

Now ask yourself, 'What's happening with me **right now?**'

1. Acknowledge

Acknowledge whatever you are experiencing in your **body**. What physical sensations are you aware of? Itching, pain, discomfort, hot, cold, clothes against your skin, the points of contact with the chair and floor? Whatever the experience is, just notice and acknowledge it.

Check in also with what is going on in your **mind**. Are you busy thinking, worrying, planning, making lists? Is your mind busy or still and empty?

Whatever is going on in your mind, the task is merely to observe it neutrally and without judgement.

Then, take your attention to how you feel **emotionally**. Happy, sad, angry, stressed, anxious, calm? Again, just notice this, not trying to change it but acknowledging that it's just how things are right now.

2. Gather
Now, from the wider awareness of body, mind and emotions, gather up all of your focus and place it deliberately on your own breathing and nothing else. Focus on the sensations of breathing from moment to moment. Follow the movement of air as it enters and leaves the body. Notice the rise and fall of the chest, the rhythmic movement of the in breath and out breath. When your mind wanders away from focusing on the breath, which it will, because that's what minds do, gently bring the focus back to the breath. We carry our breath with us wherever we go, so focusing on the breath is a way to anchor ourselves in a busy world.

3. Expand
When you feel ready, expand your focus outwards from the narrow focus on the breath to again take in an awareness of the whole body. Notice the points of contact of your body with the chair and floor. Begin to notice the sounds around you and become aware of your surroundings. When you feel ready, open your eyes.

If this short meditation had a shape, it would be like an hour-glass – wide awareness, to narrow, to wide again.

Carer organisations

Most areas have a carers association, carers centre or other kind of carer support agency, and it is very well worth finding out about your local carer organisation to explore ways they can support you. Often this may include giving advice on benefits, offering counselling, providing complementary therapies to help with carer stress, supporting working carers and possibly running regular support groups, and they are often the way that statutory organisations such as the local authority consult with carers about policy changes.

Accepting help

Community kindness was discussed in Chapter 5, but offers of help are only as good as the willingness to accept that help. Good old British pride and the 'soldier on regardless' mentality are fine while you're coping, but it then becomes hard to make that first step to say you're struggling and ask for help.

If someone offers to mow the lawn, let them, even if you can still manage to do it yourself. It's one less thing to think about. One less task to fit into busy days filled with caring. If someone offers to get your newspaper, let them, even if you could actually get it delivered. Have you guessed why? Well, when they come over to mow the lawn, drop off the paper, or the shopping or whatever, you will have a bit of a chat, and that social interaction is priceless when you are a carer for someone with advanced dementia. It will help you feel less isolated, it will lift your spirits, there will be someone who will notice if you're struggling, and it adds to the web of support around you that provides reassurance as you continue to do the best you can. There are neighbours who would be willing to help, but you 'don't like to bother them because we're private people'. I've heard it so many times. With the growing numbers of people being diagnosed with dementia, as pointed out in the Introduction, and a lack of statutory resources to cope with this increasing need, I would argue that a whole-community response is required to ensure people living with dementia and their families feel supported.

Respite care

Continuing on the theme of self-care, organising some respite care to give yourself a break is a real investment in refuelling your energy reserves to enable you to continue caring. I have met carers who are exhausted from not taking a break for years on end because they would feel guilty for putting their loved one 'in a home', even for a short period. However, respite can take many forms. I know some families whose home care package covers several time slots per week to enable the carer to go out and spend time on their own or to attend a class or enjoy their hobbies. Where possible, if the care agency can provide a consistent member of staff, this will benefit both the carer and the person living with dementia. The carer, because they will be reassured that the home carer knows their loved one well, and the person with dementia will become familiar and relaxed with a consistent person.

When it comes to going away for a few days or a holiday, the options are varied, and with planning can again be positive all round. One option would be a short stay in a care home. There are pros and cons, and there is no right or wrong answer. Care homes are experts in care, but the person with dementia will be in an unfamiliar place, which can cause them to be unsettled. If the person with dementia has a home care package, it may be possible to arrange for a relative or friend to stay with them, keeping the usual home care visits in place. Many home care agencies now also provide home respite support via 24-hour care, but this will need to be written into their care agreement and care plan, usually by a social worker, GP or dementia nurse. Whatever a carer needs to do to give themselves permission to take care of themselves and not feel judged by others for taking time out is crucial to making the experience of caring more pleasurable and less stressful.

Planning ahead

I wanted to point out here that planning ahead is yet another way to alleviate stress. It is sometimes difficult to see the need while things are ticking along okay, but then a crisis happens – a fall, a hospital admission, a carer illness – and there is no contingency in place, making a stressful event even more distressing. Such events can often prove to be the shock that pushes a carer to decide the time has come for the person with dementia to move into residential care. However, if things had been in place sooner, this could possibly be avoided or at least delayed.

Getting advice on equipment and house adaptations, advanced financial and health care decisions and thoughts about care preferences can all be in place ahead of time. We often use the analogy with people that you wouldn't set off to go on holiday abroad without your passport, packing a case, checking you had travel insurance and getting the correct currency. Therefore, why would we want to embark on a dementia journey, which will affect all aspects of our daily lives, without a plan for how to cope as needs change? A social worker, dementia nurse or one of the many charities that support people living with dementia, such as the Alzheimer's Society, can give advice on these matters.

Maintaining a carer's own sense of identity

It is so incredibly easy for a carer's sense of self to become lost to this label of 'carer'. My heart goes out to family members whose own life can seem 'on hold' as they prioritise the needs of their loved one with dementia. I hear the 'used to' so often. 'I used to enjoy going fishing, but I can't get away now.' 'We used to love foreign holidays, but he couldn't take the travel any more, which means I can't go either.' There are so many examples I could give along these lines. I can't overstate the importance of finding a way to maintain hobbies, friendships, interests, and so on, whilst not pretending that finding solutions to enable this are always easy. It is an emotion that carers do not like speaking about, but resentment towards the person with dementia is natural and is only deepened if the carer doesn't find a way to continue with aspects of their own life that are important to them.

The carer's own personality will also contribute to the interplay of the dementia caring journey, and this requires an increased level of self-awareness and self-acceptance. If a wife has always been house-proud and has a need to be in control of things, for example, it can be incredibly challenging to accept the person living with dementia making a mess or not complying with instructions. Practising a mindful pause can help. It is not a personal affront on her standards: the person with dementia can't help it, and there is no point in constantly telling them off about it and causing distress on both sides. Another example would be for a carer who has never found it easy to express how they feel about things. Being able to talk to someone and be honest about feelings may feel alien, but will be so helpful to ensure you get the support you need and deserve as a carer.

Volunteers and carers

When I first began training volunteers and establishing the home visits, my focus had been on helping people to build a connection and communicate with the person living with dementia. What became obvious very quickly was that of equal importance was the building of a trusting relationship with the carers as well.

We were getting feedback that carers were also looking forward to the Namaste Care visit, and I realised that this was also fulfilling a social and support function for the carers. I now advise volunteers to 'check in and check out' with the carers, giving them a chance to talk about anything that is on their minds. It is not the volunteer's role to find a solution for carers, but listening in itself will relieve stress and anxiety. We had hoped that carers would like to learn some of the Namaste approach from volunteer visitors, but this has happened less often than we imagined. What seems to be of more help to carers is to receive reassurance from the volunteer that they are doing a good job of caring and to use the time of the visit as a little bit of time for themselves or to get other things done that have been building up.

I recently reviewed one of our long-standing Namaste Care relationships which has been going for a year. The carer told me how he doesn't know how he would have coped without the volunteer. It would be easy to dismiss the importance of a once-weekly visit for a couple of hours by a volunteer, but to the family it clearly means a great deal that someone is taking such a close interest in their loved one. If I am honest, it brought a tear to my eye and I had incredible pride in the volunteer for her genuineness and compassion. The volunteer has been alongside the family on the final stages of the journey of dementia, and now the lady with dementia's needs are changing, she has been a steadying presence for the family and has fed back any concerns for the family via supervision, enabling support from services to be re-activated when needed. She is therefore a key link for us between family and services; but on a personal level, she has forged a truly lovely relationship with the lady she visits.

In conclusion to this chapter on carer needs, I want to state my opinion that carers are worth their weight in gold, and Namaste Care can be a way to enjoy time with and have a positive connection to the person living with dementia, enabling families to approach the end of life in a more meaningful way.

12

Sensory Stimulation

There are about one billion neurons in a human brain, creating 100 trillion synapses or connections. 'That is at least 1,000 times the number of stars in our galaxy' (Ross 2011). These are mind-boggling numbers, and I am no neuroscientist. My simplistic way to think about neural pathways is to imagine them like pathways through a forest. The ones that are used frequently become familiar, well-worn paths, whilst the less-used ones become overgrown. Very strongly wired neural pathways become habitual, and they account, for example, for those automatic journeys in a car where you end up taking the turning for work when you were intending to visit a friend in the opposite direction. In my over-simplified analogy, sensory stimulation with people living with dementia is a way of attempting to keep the pathways as well tended as possible for as long as possible, given the fact that there will be an inevitable decline due to progression of the illness.

The benefits of sensory stimulation are listed by GoldenCarers[1] as being:

- Improved cognitive symptoms and maintaining daily function

- Encouragement to participate in social groups

- Opportunities for reflection and trips down memory lane

- Increased concentration and alertness

- Facilitation of communication

I wonder if this is partly because a common reaction to a diagnosis of dementia is reduced activity, keeping safe at home, being socially isolated,

---

1   www.goldencarers.com

and a lack of stimulation. Sensory stimulation therefore redresses some of this deficit in stimulation.

The idea of using sensory stimulation started in the Netherlands in the 1960s, originally with the aim to help people with learning disabilities explore their environment. In the case of conditions such as autism, it was noticed that environments that are very busy in terms of multiple sensory stimuli can often lead to the person with autism being over-stimulated and unable to cope. Similarly, people living with dementia report becoming more sensitive to sounds and busy environments, finding it overwhelming to be in places where there are lots of things going on at once (people talking, background noise, traffic, crowds). Therefore, sensory approaches need to slow things down and not over-stimulate.

From experience of using sensory stimulation approaches, I would recommend keeping in mind the following aims. Sensory stimulation should be:

- Gentle

- Enjoyable

- Relaxing

- Simple

- Creative

Putting it into practice

Now let's explore in a little more detail how it can be done. The Canadian Association of Occupational Therapists recommends the use of everyday, familiar objects with a focus on one or two senses at a time. This turns everyday items such as a hairbrush, autumn leaves, clothing and favourite foods into sensory cues. These are presented to the person one at a time, with each stimulus used as a focus for chatting about memories or about the wellbeing of the person living with dementia. As Alzheimers.net describe it, 'Sensory stimulation uses everyday objects to arouse one or more of the five senses (hearing, sight, smell, taste and touch), with the goal of evoking positive feelings' (Alzheimers.net 2017).

Let me give you a practical example. If I massaged the hands of someone who has worked as a typist, I would comment on how much hard work these hands have done in their lifetime and wonder whether the person's hands ever got tired or ached. I might bring up a memory that I have found out from the Life Story, or I could comment on how the person has beautiful skin or long, elegant fingers. You can therefore see some underlying principles of Namaste Care at work here:

- Honouring who the person is and has been in their life

- Promoting good self-esteem

- Enhancing a positive mood

- Attending to the person's wellbeing

So, always attempting to link activities to the person's interests in life, the following are some examples of activities that could be tried out.

Smell

- Scented room spritz

- Favourite perfume or aftershave

- Scented massage cream/wax/lotion

- Soap

- Flowers and herbs

- Aromatherapy diffuser

- Cooking smells – bread, toast, curry, etc. (combined then with tasting)

Sight

- Old photographs

- Books with illustrations

- Flowers/seasonal items

- What you wear (such as wearing a forties or fifties outfit to visit the person)

- Going outside

- Gardening (combines with smell and touch)

- DVDs (musicals, old comedy shows, relaxing nature films)

- Blowing bubbles
- Antique items (everyday items used by the person, such as a rolling pin or typewriter, for example)
- Exploring items related to a hobby (such as football memorabilia)

Sound

- Favourite music (create a playlist from the person's teens, early twenties and significant events)
- Musical instruments
- Rainmaker
- Reading aloud
- Wind chimes
- Radio (if appropriate and not confusing with too many adverts and chat)

Taste

- Favourite treats
- Drinks
- Sensory baking
- Related to the season or a theme

Touch

- Hand, foot or scalp massage
- Applying face cream
- Hand and feet washing
- Hand holding
- Fiddle mitts/blankets
- Seasonal items such as acorns in autumn, sand to reminisce about family holidays, etc.

- Fabrics – varied types (e.g. lace, satin, cotton)

- Hair brushing and styling

- Soothing bath

- Applying make-up or nail varnish

In a systematic review of research into non-pharmacological interventions, which aimed to reduce agitation in people living with dementia, the only interactions found by Kong *et al.* (2009) to have a moderate degree of effectiveness were sensory interactions. Specifically listed were the following:

- Calming music

- Aromatherapy

- Thermal baths

- Hand massages

Given these findings, and based on our own experiences within the project of what works well, let us focus on these areas in a little more detail.

Music

Imagine what the soundtrack to your life would be. Take a moment to think about it. From being in the womb we will most likely have been hearing music, the most basic of which was our mother's heartbeat. But we would also be hearing the radio, the TV, any music those around us chose to play. Then once we're born we are surrounded by sounds. Our parents may have played their favourite music, we would watch children's TV and hear theme tunes, advert jingles and musicals. Through our teens we develop our own taste in music, often tinged with teenage angst and first-love experiences. A strong musical memory for me would be all the musicals I took part in during school and the choir songs we learned. Rehearsing over and over learned lyrics and tunes leads to a strong neural pathway, and I still remember the words to all the songs in *Oklahoma*. I sang them to my children when they were young, so now they remember them too.

Then there is music with a special meaning, such as the music that was playing when you met your partner or the song you and your friends always danced to when it was played. Mine is 'Summer of '69' by Bryan Adams, but everyone's will be era-specific and personal-taste-specific. There's the first dance at your wedding, music that reminds you of a loss, music that reminds you of a holiday, and so on. The moment you hear a piece of music it will transport you back to a time and memory that is associated with that music. Music can calm us, stir our emotions, make us cry, make us joyful. So, imagine the potential for using music to help someone living with dementia to honour who they are and to respect their personal preferences and loves.

In 2018, staff at Her Majesty's Passport Office, Durham, raised money for the Namaste Care Project, after hearing about our work when I gave a presentation to their Carers Conference. Namaste Care never fails to touch people's hearts. We used the money they raised to buy in some amazing training for our staff and volunteers at the hospice from a charity called Playlist for Life.

Playlist for Life was founded by Sally Magnusson (writer, broadcaster and daughter of Magnus Magnusson) in 2013 after the death of her mother Mamie. Mamie had been cared for at home by her family after developing dementia, and the family noted that no matter how much symptoms progressed, they could still reach Mamie through music. She could remember the words to songs long after she could no longer have a conversation. They noted that Mamie was more alert after listening to music, and in Sally's own words quoted in the Playlist for Life training manual: 'Music more than anything else was keeping my mother with us.'

As was explained to us in the training: 'Music, emotion and autobiographical memories come together in an area of the brain called the pre-frontal cortex. And as we have already explained, music connects with many parts of the brain.' This means that if one part of the brain is damaged by dementia, music will stimulate other parts.

The training encourages us to become 'Music Detectives' and to put together a personal playlist of music that is meaningful to each individual living with dementia. Ideas for music to consider are in the following areas:

- Songs and artists linked to childhood (school songs, family songs, lullabies, TV theme tunes)
- Favourite bands, singers and shows
- Dance music
- Songs related to special memories
- Wedding songs (first dance, for example)
- Songs related to holidays

- Christmas and seasonal songs

- Songs from a particular era, especially the person's teen years (war songs and fifties and sixties albums, for example)

It is worth also finding out whether the person played an instrument. They may still be able to.

How the music is played will very much depend on personal circumstances. For comfort, an MP3 player is best used with over-the-ear headphones rather than ear buds, and this may be the best solution if the person is sharing space with others who don't want to listen to the same music. Otherwise CD players, music DVDs, radio and so on could all be tried.

If it is not known what type of music the person would enjoy, relaxing music and nature sounds have been shown to have a calming and stress-reducing effect.

Aromatherapy

Using aromatherapy offers both an opportunity and a caution, but first it is worth exploring a little about the background of aromatherapy.

> Aromatherapy is the use of therapeutic oils extracted from natural plant matter in order to encourage good health, equilibrium and wellbeing. The essential oils that are used in aromatherapy are truly holistic in that they can have a powerful and positive effect on mind, body and spirit. (Walters 1998)

There are many references to the use of essential oils across history. The Ancient Egyptians clearly explored uses of plant essences for perfume, embalming and ceremonial use. In Ancient Greece, Hippocrates, considered to be the 'Father of Medicine', mentions a vast number of plant uses in his many works, and many other pioneering historical figures built on his work.

Famous Roman writers have been influential, such as Pliny the Elder (AD23–79), with his many botanical references in his major work, *Historia Naturalis*, or the Roman physician Galen (AD129–200), who studied and observed the effects of plant use in order to produce a diagnosis and prognosis. Uses of herbs and essences continued to be explored through the centuries, with Nicholas Culpeper being a great herbalist of his day in the 17th century.

However, it could be argued that the French chemist René-Maurice Gattefossé was the most influential figure in the shape that *modern aromatherapy* has taken, as it was he who first used the term 'aromatherapie' in 1926 after his famous accidental discovery of the healing power of lavender on his burns. As a chemist, he was able to understand that the antiseptic and healing properties of lavender were far superior to any synthetic chemical, which had become more commonly used in medicine through the 19th and early 20th centuries.

Following this discovery (or rediscovery), the interest in essences rapidly grew for use in cosmetics, and another Frenchman, Dr Valnet, further developed research in this area during his time as a surgeon in the Second World War when medical supplies were short. Valnet's scientific approach and resulting data, as well as his dedication to share his findings on the use of essences, which was started by Gattefossé, provide the foundation for aromatherapy today.

Essential oils can enter the body either through inhalation or being absorbed through the skin. They enter the blood stream and have an effect on the body's limbic system. The limbic system is a very ancient part of human evolution and is where our instincts, memories and basic vital functions and responses are controlled. The limbic system will register the presence of an aroma molecule and release chemicals in response, either to calm the body or to stimulate it to action. So if we smell something that is associated with a trauma, our body will respond with alarm and develop a stress response. Whereas if the limbic system detects a smell associated with calm and safety, then the body will relax and there will be a sense of wellbeing.

So here lies an opportunity, but there are also cautions. Let's deal with the cautions first before looking at the positive ways to use aromatherapy.

A question that we ask in the Life Story is about any smells that might bring back a bad memory. The family may know this information, but not always, so it is never possible to totally rule out all potential negative responses. We can just do the best we can to find out. One lady we completed a Life Story with associated the smell of furniture polish with a very scary grandmother. Another associated the smell of lemons with death. A lovely gentleman had an accident resulting in burns from a bonfire, so Guy Fawkes Night in the UK and the smell of open fires was always tricky for him (as described in Chapter 8). Knowing this, if we can, is really useful in informing our Namaste Care approach.

With regard to using essential oils, we do have to be cautious, given their effects on the body. Any individual essential oil *must not be used undiluted*. It must be diluted in a carrier oil or other medium and should only be prescribed and blended by a qualified aromatherapist. Care must also be taken with sun exposure following the application of essential oils, as many of them can create photosensitivity on the skin. They need to be stored away from direct sunlight in a cool, dry place and may have a use-by date which should be checked.

In covering the cautions, however, I do not seek to put people off using this wonderful therapy. There are ways to use essential oils safely that will benefit people living with dementia. For example, I associate the smell of rose with my lovely grandma. I remember snuggles with her in front of the fire, a sense of safety and being loved and her gentle, funny ways. I tend to prefer rose-based perfume, soap, cut flowers and face cream, obviously in response to these positive associations. This is something my family could continue for me if I develop dementia.

With regard to safe use of essential oils, it is best to buy pre-blended oils to avoid the necessity of mixing them ourselves. Purchasing a pre-blended massage oil for 'relaxation' or 'soothing' or 'stress relief' or 'uplifting' gets around the issue of needing an aromatherapist to prescribe and blend for you. If you look at the ingredients, you will find that many will be blended in an oil such as sweet almond (so check for nut allergies) or grapeseed oil and will use one, two or three essential oils to create the desired effect. Here are some common essential oils with their main benefits:

- Lavender – relaxing, calming, good for encouraging sleep

- Lemongrass – anti-depressant, stimulating

- Neroli – soothing to the nerves, anti-depressant

- Chamomile – comforting and healing

- Ylang-Ylang – soothing, lowers blood pressure

- Frankincense – uplifting and spiritual

- Mandarin – stimulating and balancing

- Rose – balancing and uplifting

- Geranium – cheerful and balancing

If I were to recommend one essential oil above all others, I would suggest using lemon balm (Melissa officinalis) as there is a growing body of evidence about its safety and usefulness for people living with a dementia. Lemon balm has been shown to have a calming but *not* sedative effect, unlike lavender which is sedative. It has been shown in clinical trials (Ballard *et al.* 2002) to enhance mood and quality of life when compared to a placebo. As with all essential oils, it needs to be a good quality oil and diluted in a carrier oil for massage or added to water in a diffuser. Joyce Simard notes:

> Aromatherapy and the use of essential oils – especially lavender, geranium and marjoram – may have calming effects on anxious residents (Flanagan 1995). However, these oils should not be used on any resident with allergies. Aromatherapy is a natural, non-invasive treatment system. It has been observed that the aroma of lavender in the Namaste Care room appears to create a calming environment and may be one of the reasons why pacing residents are drawn into the room to sit and rest. (Simard 2013)

Using aromatherapy is such a positive benefit to people living with dementia that it is worth exploring its use within the home. Aromatherapy diffusers and scented room spritzes are widely available now from many outlets, and the family will also gain the benefit of this fragrant and calming intervention.

Thermal baths

For many people with advanced dementia, having a bath becomes a thing of the past due to issues with not being able to physically get into a bath. Most people we work with use a shower chair in a wet room or walk-in shower due to mobility issues. So, although research tells us that thermal baths are very therapeutic and relaxing, it can be easier said than done when people are living at home.

One lady we had been working with came into the hospice for end-of-life care, and while in her last week of life, the hospice staff carefully and lovingly hoisted her into our special whirlpool bath and apparently the look on her face was blissful as she curled herself up in the warm, soothing water. Some residential homes will have the ability to offer baths to residents, and even some people living at home may have adaptations that enable people to continue having baths. A bath is a lovely, relaxing way to offer a sensory experience with the addition of beautiful scented bath products, and the warm water will help to ease aching joints and stiff muscles, providing pain relief and whole body relaxation.

However, in the spirit of Namaste Care, we work with the environment we have and do the best we can. So if there isn't the option to offer someone a relaxing bath, we need to explore ways to make their shower or bed bath the most beautiful, caring experience it can possibly be. It is easy for a shower or bed bath to become just another care task to get out of the way, but if we adopt this attitude, we are missing an opportunity to enhance the person's sensory experiences. So, when helping the person with a shower, we could use lovely, luxurious scented shower gels or jellies, or we could use a natural sponge or a loofah to add a tactile sensation to the experience. We could take our time and let the person really relax into and enjoy the experience. The addition of mood lighting and colour-changing light units can enhance the sensory environment. With a little thought, we can create a sensory experience out of a mundane care task. We could also take a bowl of warm, scented water to the person to wash their hands, face or feet, or indeed use warm flannels to wash them and give them a pleasant sensory cleanse.

Similarly with a bed bath, giving some thought to the products used to bath the person, wrapping them in warm towels afterwards and using scented lotions and creams afterwards all add to the person's daily quality of life.

Hand massages

Offering a person living with dementia a hand, foot or scalp massage is such a fundamental part of Namaste Care that I have devoted the next chapter entirely to an exploration of loving touch. Suffice to say here that a hand massage is a simple yet powerful way to build trust and connection in a non-verbal way with someone in the advanced stages of dementia. We would always offer a massage skin to skin (without gloves) unless there is an infection-control issue.

Enriching the environment

Luke Tanner (2017) reminds us that we can give thought to how we enrich the care environment so that there are plenty of opportunities for sensory stimulation within easy reach of the person living with dementia. This does not mean filling the space around a person with a chaotic array of 'stuff' but giving careful thought to what would be personally meaningful to them in an advanced stage of dementia.

> For someone experiencing the late stages of dementia, being in touch with things means holding, grasping, touching, feeling, tapping, shaking, hugging and stroking things. This is more about the sensory stimulation that such items offer and can be a way for someone to shape the way they feel. (Tanner 2017)

Thinking about objects that relate to the person's life history can help to restore a sense of self, and they are easier for a person with late-stage dementia to relate to than representational communication such as verbal language or pictures. 'Without any stuff to hand that is familiar there are no familiar sensations' (Tanner 2017). Familiarity breeds a feeling of safety and reassurance, so a memory box of personal sensory items can be a very powerful resource.

Brain plasticity – hints of something exciting?

In concluding this chapter on sensory stimulation, I wanted to mention an area that may offer some hope for how we care for people with dementia and how we might approach their care. Our project has shown us the glimpse of something exciting. One lady, after 16 visits from her volunteer, remembered and used her name. Another lady began to anticipate her foot massage by taking her socks off when the volunteer came. People with dementia aren't meant to be able to learn and retain new things, and yet…

Due to the ability of the brain to re-wire itself, an ability that persists into old age, it is possible for people to be rehabilitated following brain damage caused by stroke, an accident or other kinds of brain injury. 'The adult brain is not entirely "hard wired" with fixed neuronal circuits. There are many instances of cortical and subcortical rewiring of neuronal circuits in response to training as well as in response to injury.'[2]

I am not for one minute suggesting we could cure or even substantially rehabilitate the brain of someone with dementia. Dementia is a progressive condition and we still have an awful lot to learn about it. However, there does seem to be the possibility of some sensory benefit to a repeated, positive and loving experience, in familiar, relaxed surroundings, that appears to enhance the cognitive function even very slightly and temporarily as a result of Namaste Care. If we structure the Namaste Care sessions the same each time we visit, could this visit become a positive ritual? Much more research is needed, and maybe there is scope for the development of some more kinds of cognitive therapy techniques.

---

2   https://en.m.wikipedia.org/wiki/neuroplasticity

13

Loving Touch

The power of loving touch is the foundation of Namaste Care and becomes the thread that weaves the fabric of the day to create a cocoon of love for the residents we care for and care about.

Joyce Simard 2013

No particular sense is more important than another, but in terms of building a relationship between two people, the sense of touch links people physically, spiritually and emotionally. It is therefore a powerful tool to create soothing, safety and connection if used in an intentionally loving and caring way. Joyce Simard reminds us that touch is communication and can accompany a greeting, can provide gentle guidance and is above all a universal form of reassurance when used with a soothing and encouraging tone of voice and facial expression.

There is evidence that from ancient times human beings understood the importance of physical touch and the therapeutic benefits it has for the body and mind. From Ancient China to Ancient Greece, the holistic view of health involves touch therapies in some form or another.

In early life, the amount of loving touch we receive can literally shape our brains. Touch helps us to deal with stress, boosts our immune system and builds attachments to loved ones. As Sue Gerhardt expresses it in her book *Why Love Matters*:

> When we are physically held, we know that we are supported by others. There is a moment in Ashley Montague's film, *Touching*, which conveys this movingly: a distraught and distracted patient in a mental hospital, being interviewed by a psychiatrist, seems much more able to focus on the psychiatrist's face and engage with him when the psychiatrist reaches out and grasps his hand

to convey his concern for the patient. These deep satisfactions of touch remain part of adult life, as bereaved people are comforted by a hug, partners communicate how 'in touch' they are with each other sexually, or people let go of the stresses of their daily life with a massage. (Gerhardt 2004)

An important aspect of Namaste Care is therefore offering a gentle hand and foot massage as a way to connect with a person living with dementia that does not require words. Massage releases the hormone oxytocin, which is associated with feelings of safety and love, so we can directly improve the quality of life for someone living with dementia with this simple act of kindness.

Massage as a technique has its origins in a caring caress – after an injury, we rub the area that is in pain, while parents tell their children to 'rub it better' when they hurt themselves. Dogs lick themselves when they have an injury. The therapeutic value of touch has a place in all aspects of healthcare. (Norris 2012)

In summary, the benefits of a gentle massage could include that it is:

- Comforting – known to reduce stress and relax muscles

- Communicative – allows us to connect without the need for words

- Instinctive – we naturally reach out to comfort someone who is distressed or in pain

- Stimulating – improves circulation and helps prevent muscle stiffness

- Relaxing – helps prevent muscle stiffness and soothes aches and pains

- Safe – non-threatening and non-invasive

- Mutual – both the giver and receiver of the massage will feel the relaxing effect

Ethical considerations

As with everything we seek to do with someone living with dementia, gaining consent may need to be approached more broadly. Our referral forms ask if there is any reason why this person should not have a gentle hand and foot massage, and so we are introducing this element of the care early on. I also write to GPs to let them know that the person living with dementia is going to be having Namaste Care visits and ask them to let me know if there are any reasons they should not have a hand and foot massage. We use consent forms (see Appendix), which the main carer can sign if the person with dementia is unable to sign on their own behalf. On another practical note, all of our volunteers are DBS-checked, given that they will be spending one-to-one time with a vulnerable adult and engaging in loving touch.

However, these procedures are administrative and are in a way an abstract concept to try to convey. Some people living with dementia have never had a massage before, and so there is no substitute for showing them directly by giving them a short hand massage and observing their response. A person living with dementia can demonstrate very clearly by their actions of pulling away, facial expression and a shake of the head that they do not want a massage, and we would respect this clear signal. This type of rejection of touch is very uncommon and may just be a reflection of how the person is feeling that particular day. So trying again on other days is always worth it. More often the touch through massage is welcomed and enjoyed.

Indeed, loving touch has been shown to decrease the likelihood of a rejection of care. In situations where someone living with dementia has been labelled as aggressive or non-co-operative with care tasks, this can lead to a negative cycle of fear on both sides and deterioration in relationships. However, Ladislav Volicer notes the power of loving touch:

> Loving touch approach decreases rejection of care because residents are exposed to loving touch repeatedly during Namaste Care session. This experience makes them more tactile; more accepting of being touched and this tolerance transfers also to touch necessary for provision of care. (Volicer 2015)

As a result of introducing loving touch approaches through Namaste Care, care homes note residents are less resistive to care, they complain less about pain during care tasks, and the staff team feel more satisfied and less stressed in their job.

We could conclude therefore that, ethically, loving touch is a benefit and will improve quality of life. It is generally accepted as a positive approach and is something anyone can do (family, friends, paid carers) to assist the person living with dementia feel settled and connected to others.

Ways to provide loving touch

There are a number of very natural and everyday ways to touch someone appropriately and with tender, loving care. There are few things more glorious than someone gently and slowly brushing your hair (whether you have hair or not, Joyce Simard would point out). So here are some ideas for touch that could be tried:

- Hair combing, brushing and styling (men often used Brylcreem in the past)

- Lovingly washing face, hands and feet

- Dancing together (if mobility allows)

- Applying face cream (such as Pond's cold cream for reminiscence or aftershave for men)

- Hugs around the shoulders

- Manicures/nail filing/applying nail varnish

- Hand-over-hand guidance during an activity

- Hand holding or a handshake

- Hand, scalp and foot massages

Massage

So, now let's focus in on massage in particular as something that can be seen as a core activity in Namaste Care.

Safety

I always do a patch test on the forearm with a small amount of the massage oil, cream or wax to be used, usually on my first or second visit, to check for reactions. Generally, if someone has sensitive skin, this will already be known, and in many cases we can then use their own emollient or moisturising cream to avoid any unwanted skin reactions.

Instances when massage is *not* recommended would be:

- over an open wound or fracture site

- when the person has medical lymphedema (this requires treatment by a specialist)

- if the person has a systemic infection making them feel unwell

- when the person has a skin infection that could be spread

- when the person giving the massage has any kind of contagious infection

- directly over a tumour site

- if the person has a deep vein thrombosis

- after a recent injury or over bruised areas.

Other situations where *caution is needed* and medical advice should be sought include the following conditions:

- Osteoporosis

- Altered skin sensation

- When taking blood-thinning medication

- Circulatory conditions

Given that the type of massage recommended for people living with dementia is very light touch, it may be suitable despite the cautions, but it is always worth checking it out.

Thought should also be given to the psychological and behavioural aspects of each person living with dementia, and this is where good knowledge about their background is so helpful. For example, if the person has a history of physical or sexual abuse, they may be especially frightened or intolerant of touch. In this situation, we would approach with care and nurturing to see if the appropriate touch of a hand massage was welcomed, and to avoid misinterpretation, it may be beneficial to be in the presence of a third party to provide extra reassurance.

In terms of potential behaviour, at times a person living with dementia may become frustrated, agitated, tired, aggressive and restless. While a gentle hand massage is most likely to soothe a person, the individual giving the massage must also keep themselves safe and not force the issue. The person may be experiencing delusions or paranoia, which makes approaching them unhelpful at that time. Knowing the person, observing them and respecting their space when they appear to be unreceptive to touch will build trust, in that you are demonstrating that you understand their needs and this will hopefully strengthen any relationship still further. You can then attempt to connect through touch at a more conducive time for the person.

Preparing for massage

You do not need to be qualified in massage to give a gentle and safe hand massage. Very little equipment is required and, with the right intention, it is a gorgeous way to feel close to someone and demonstrate how much they are valued and cared for.

One thing to consider is the type of massage medium that will be appropriate to use. Here is a brief guide to what is available:

- **Massage oils** – probably the most widely used massage medium is plant-based oil. Grapeseed oil is cheap but is slightly astringent, so may not be the best choice for very dry skin. An oil like evening primrose, sweet almond (so long as there is not a nut allergy issue) or jojoba is more nourishing to the skin but can be more expensive.

- **Massage gels** – these are water-based substances and are non-oily, so leave no residue. These are a good choice if the person likes to feel less oily or has very oily skin. Some contain herbal blends, which can be therapeutic, such as a lavender gel or aloe vera. Gels can be soothing and cooling on a hot day, but they are absorbed rapidly, so may not be suitable for someone with dry skin.

- **Massage creams** – good for small areas such as the hands or face and are excellent for very dry skin due to having high oil content. They can be absorbed readily, so may need more frequent application.

- **Hand lotions and creams** – widely available and can be used for massage, but some use less natural ingredients and require more frequent application.

- **Massage powders** – great for a person who does not like the sensation of oil on the skin or if they are very hairy or have very oily skin.

- **Massage waxes** – a solid that turns to oil on contact with the body. This is what we use in our project following a recommendation by St Joseph's Hospice in Hackney, London. We use 'Songbird' massage waxes, available online, which have lovely essential oil blends added to give the extra therapeutic benefit and a wonderful smell.

- **Prescription creams** – we have often worked with people who have emollient creams prescribed, either due to allergy or dry skin conditions. In this situation we would use the person's own cream for the massage.

Massage media should be stored in a cool, dry cupboard and expiry dates checked before use. The only other equipment required is a pillow, a towel and some relaxing music.

Ensuring that the person living with dementia is seated well, ideally slightly reclined with all of their body supported, will allow them to relax fully during the massage. There is no hard and fast rule about when to offer the massage. This can be led by the person with dementia. For example, if the person was unsettled and agitated at the beginning of a Namaste visit, it may be most appropriate to start with a gentle washing of the hands and a hand massage to soothe the person and to connect with them. However, if the person is quite sleepy already, it may be more appropriate to start with more stimulating activities and then end with the massage.

The other consideration for giving a massage is our own posture and ensuring we are in a comfortable seating position with our back aligned and upright so that we do not hurt ourselves or become uncomfortable midway through the massage. Sitting at the same height, not having to reach too far and removing any rings and watches beforehand will ensure that the massage can go ahead uninterrupted.

I find for myself, and volunteers also tell me, that it is incredibly calming and therapeutic to give a massage, so there is a win-win benefit to this delightful activity. Often volunteers are timid about trying it in training in case they 'do it wrong' but quickly come to love this activity as a core activity for Namaste Care.

Suggested massage approach – The 'M Technique'

It is very difficult to go wrong with a hand massage, other than applying too much pressure or not considering the cautions above. Over the small area of the lower arm and hand, the main massage moves would consist of:

- Stroking – using the whole palm or the thumbs to stroke over an area

- Circling – using the thumbs to circle over the skin, especially over the small joints in the hand

- Gentle pulling and pressing – pulling down the fingers, for example, and pressing the tips

The M Technique is a simple approach to giving a hand massage that recommends doing everything three times. The first time it is new, the second time it's familiar and the third time you know it. This builds trust and allows the body to relax because it recognises the pattern and rhythm and knows what to expect. Also we can use three as a measure of pressure, so if zero was no pressure and 10 was crushing pressure, we would use a pressure of about 3, guided by the verbal or non-verbal feedback of the person receiving the massage.[1]

A summary of a suggested routine is as follows, but it is fine to develop your own and to just enjoy the experience together.

- Ensure you have washed your hands prior to starting.

- Make initial contact by holding the person's hand, smiling and making eye contact, then explaining what you are about to do.

- Apply some massage medium to your own hands and then begin with three slow strokes with the palm of your hand up from the person's hand to their elbow. Repeat this three times.

- Circle the elbow joint three times with your thumbs.

- Make small circles three times around the wrist bones.

- Placing your hands either side of the person with dementia's hand, using both thumbs, stroke outwards from the centre of the hand to the outside, starting at the wrist and working down to the knuckles. Repeat three times.

- Using thumbs, circle each joint in the hand three times from the knuckle down each finger. To finish each finger, grasp the finger gently and pull down the finger with a cupped hand, then apply a small amount of pressure to the fingertip where there is a pressure point.

- If the person with dementia is able to, turn the hand over and stroke across the palm using the thumbs three times.

- Finish with the same move used to start, sweeping up to the elbow with your palm three times.

- End by holding the person's hand and smiling.

- Use the towel to remove any excess oil from that hand and then wrap it in one side of the towel to keep it warm, while you move across to the other hand and repeat the process.

---

1   An excellent demonstration of the technique from St Michael's Hospice, by Beatrice Veal, is available at www.youtube.com/watch?v=OfZxM6jTr9s

Foot massages are also incredibly relaxing, often sending people off to sleep; however, there are a few more issues to consider here. Some people don't like their feet being touched. I heard a story of a nurse who was kicked in the face when she tried to touch a patient's foot. Feet are much more prone to fungal infections, which could be transmitted during massage. There are also a lot of pressure points in the feet, which a qualified reflexologist will know how to work with. This said, keeping a foot massage to light pressure (if there are no infection-control issues and it is accepted by the person with dementia) is a further way to enjoy some loving touch.

The fundamental nature of touch in relationships makes it a key feature of Namaste Care. For a more in-depth consideration of issues relating to touch in care services, I would recommend Luke Tanner's book *Embracing Touch in Dementia Care: A Person-Centred Approach to Touch and Relationships* (2017). He takes apart and examines the misguided concept that it is 'unprofessional' to offer hugs and loving touch, whilst being sensitive to people's individual needs as unique and varied.

In concluding this chapter I would remind readers of the heart-breaking scenes in Romanian orphanages we saw on the TV years ago where children had been deprived of touch and this had resulted in developmental and psychological problems. Touch is part of who we are as humans, as social animals who crave connection to others. Dementia does not change this need, and we can continue to honour it as part of our care for someone living with dementia.

14

Communication

Being able to communicate is a feature of being alive. It is not only the privilege of being human, but all animals and plants have their ways to communicate. Communication is life, and we continue to communicate until we die. The gradual loss of verbal communication is one of the most distressing parts of the dementia journey. The person living with dementia experiences frustration at not being able to find the words to express themselves, and their family feel a progressive loss and worry about how to continue to communicate with them. In the advanced stages of dementia, we really do need to be willing to step into the world of the person living with dementia, rather than expecting them to fit into ours or continue to do the things they used to. Embracing this new reality can be daunting but rewarding.

As dementia progresses there are fewer attempts by carers to communicate with the person living with dementia (Kitwood 1997). This leads to the further lowering of self-esteem and withdrawal of the person with dementia, making them seem unreachable. This will place an added strain on family relationships and will impact on the quality of life of all concerned.

An often-quoted percentage for the amount of verbal communication we actually use in interactions is 7 per cent. This figure came from research by Dr Albert Mehrabian (1971) where he subtracted the voice content of interactions from all other elements. He found 38 per cent involved vocal elements such as tone of voice, and 55 per cent was expressed through non-verbal body language such as facial expression, gestures, posture, etc., giving a figure of 93 per cent of communication being non-verbal. There has been much debate about the accuracy of these statistics, but it is generally accepted that the largest proportion of communication is non-verbal. So, while we may mourn the loss of verbal communication in someone living with dementia, we should never believe that this means they can't communicate with us.

My lovely Dorothy has probably said only a handful of words to me in the time I have been visiting her due to her particular type of dementia, and yet she clearly expresses to me her likes and dislikes, and her moods; she listens to me and responds with slight movements and facial expressions. One example would be at the end of a visit when I was reading a poem to her about going to the cinema. In the poem was a list of old film star names, and when I got to Marlon Brando, her eyes widened and she began to nod her head. When I asked her husband about this, he said that Marlon Brando had been her favourite movie star. She had told me this very clearly, without the need for words.

Whilst every person living with dementia will have a different experience of their condition and their needs will change uniquely, there are some general suggestions which can help to enhance communication at an advanced stage of dementia:

- Avoid distractions and noise in order to help the person focus their attention on you.

- Be aware that your mood and attitude will affect the person with dementia, so be mindful of using relaxed, calm, respectful body language and tone of voice. Lots of smiles and reassurance will help the person to feel at ease.

- Be on the same level as the person and gain eye contact.

- Use the person's name and identify yourself by name. Joyce Simard advocates using large print name badges, as the person's ability to read was learned young and may well still be retained.

- Establish a connection by gentle touch, either holding a hand or the upper arm (which is a safe, non-threatening area of the body for touch).

- Use simple, short sentences, speaking slowly and clearly. Avoid 'chattering' as this can be too much for the person to take in.

- Avoid complicated or open-ended questions. It is better to start with yes–no choice questions and to be patient in waiting for an answer. The answer may come in a non-verbal form, so listening with our eyes as well as our ears will help with the communication.

- Remain empathic and understanding, being prepared to adjust how you are communicating according to the needs of the person.

People living with dementia can get tired easily and their ability to communicate will fluctuate throughout the day, so respecting this will enable the communication to be the most successful.

- Break down activities into steps and explain each step as you go along so the person is aware what will happen next.

- If the person with dementia becomes upset or frustrated, then acknowledge their feelings and suggest a change of subject or environment in order to distract them. 'Let's put some music on for a while.' 'Let's open the window and let some fresh air in.' 'Let's have a cup of tea.'

- Never try to convince a person with dementia they are wrong or scold them because they have forgotten something.

- Focus on long-term memories from childhood and early adulthood, as these are more likely still to be intact.

- Use singing to stimulate someone. Even when people with dementia have stopped speaking, they can still sing along to a familiar tune.

- Find out if the person seems to have a dominant sense. Often touch becomes more and more important as vision, hearing and sense of smell alter as we age.

- Use humour and try to raise a smile. The humour must never be at the person's expense, but people with dementia will often retain the social skill of laughing along with someone or finding something funny.

- Use realistic dolls and toy animals to help the person with dementia to express themselves and provide comfort.

The most important thing you will be communicating to the person by trying different ways to interact is that they still have value, they are still important and loved by their family and you are not avoiding them because you feel awkward or unsure. It is also worth exploring at this point some specific techniques that have been developed to help people with advanced dementia to communicate.

Validation Therapy

During my induction at St Cuthbert's Hospice, Sharron Tolman showed a short film of Naomi Feil, founder of Validation Therapy, working with Gladys Wilson, an 87-year-old lady living with advanced dementia (referred to by Barbara Edwards in Chapter 6). I cried. A lot of people cry when they see this film. It has captured a moment where someone who appears lost and unresponsive is once again connected and interacting meaningfully. It's a moment where the layers of dementia are peeled away and the essence of the person emerges and dances in the sunlight with you. Please watch the film[1] and have the tissues ready.

I recognised immediately what Naomi Feil was doing. It is expressing unconditional positive regard for another human being with a firm intention to connect and value the person with dementia and a willingness to step into their world.

Validation Therapy (Feil and De Klerk-Rubin 2012) is a simple but powerful approach. In summary the approach acknowledges the following:

- When we ignore difficult feelings, they gain strength. When we acknowledge these feelings, they lose their strength.

- Well-established early memories tend to stay with a person.

- Validation therapy *is not* sympathy, confrontation, distraction or reassurance. It is not patronising, but it *is* a deep empathy and understanding for a person's reality.

- Before working with someone in this way, we need to centre and ground ourselves, as it can be emotional and moving to connect with someone in this way.

- A key way to connect is to get close and make eye contact.

- Humans have many levels of consciousness and we will need to learn the person's preferred way to connect. It may be through a preferred sense or through memories, it may be through noticing and reflecting what happens in the present moment. Naomi Feil talks about 'taking the emotional temperature' of a person and naming their emotion with the same emotion.

- Touch is important, as well as noticing movement and relating to a need the person is expressing.

---

1   The short film 'Gladys Wilson and Naomi Feil' is available on YouTube at www.youtube.com/watch?v=CrZXz10FcVM

- Music that is important to the person is a powerful way to connect, as well as mirroring their movements, body language and sounds.

- The debate about whether to tell someone a 'therapeutic lie' becomes irrelevant when you embrace their reality. In this situation, telling someone every day that their mother died ten years ago when they call out for their mother would become 'You want your mother'. Constantly correcting and contradicting a person living with dementia is devaluing them and undermining their self-esteem. Calling out for mother may be a cry for comfort and love, not a mistake or 'difficult behaviour'.

Research on Validation Therapy has shown increased communication, improved mood, reduced aggressive behaviour and less need for psychotropic medications. Care workers and carers also feel more confident to handle difficult situations and feel more pleasure in their work (Tondi *et al.* 2007).

For me, acknowledging another person's reality is a basic way to show them respect and to honour their experience. Giving someone your full attention and time values them as an individual with a rich life history, one that you are interested in and care about. By not giving individuals time, a care worker designates another human being merely as an anonymous task to do and not a unique person, with needs that go beyond basic physical care. We all also have emotional and spiritual needs, right up until we take our last breath. Joyce Simard was incredibly inspired by Validation Therapy, after attending one of Naomi Feil's workshops (Simard 2013), and the influence of this approach to communicating with someone with advanced dementia is woven into the ethos of Namaste Care, which builds on the approach to include more sensory detail.

Adaptive Interaction

Another way to build and maintain close relationships with a person who is using no verbal communication is through an approach called Adaptive Interaction. Maggie Ellis and Arlene Astell (2008, 2011) have taken a technique originally developed for people with severe learning disabilities called Intensive Interaction and researched its applications for engaging people with advanced dementia. Intensive Interaction is a way of 'learning the language' of non-verbal people and using a person's communication repertoire to co-create a non-verbal conversation (Caldwell 2005).

I hear a lot that 'Bill can't communicate any more' or 'Gladys has lost her ability to communicate'. What they mean is, they have lost their ability to speak. Ellis and Astell, however, maintain that, right up until the end of our lives, we retain the communication skills we came into the world with. Babies are not born being able to speak, and yet we would never say that a baby is not communicating. They pull faces, make sounds, move and make eye contact. When you watch someone holding a baby, they will watch that baby for cues and often mirror the facial expressions and sounds back to the baby intuitively. Adaptive Interaction uses this same approach, whilst not infantilising the person living with dementia at all. The aim is to show value to how that person is communicating by reflecting it back or mirroring body movements, matching sounds and following eye gaze, so that you are essentially speaking their language.

In studies conducted in a nursing home, Ellis and Astell were able to show turn-taking behaviour, copying and a willingness to interact, resulting in smiles, laughs and an ability to express emotion. It does not allow for the expression of a specific message, but it does provide a way to connect and interact meaningfully with the person living with advanced dementia. In my experience, the biggest barrier to using this approach is people feeling self-conscious about it, but that is our hang-up to get over. If we genuinely want to enter the world of someone who is no longer using verbal communication, this is one way to do it.

Talking Mats

Developed by speech and language therapists from the University of Stirling, Talking Mats uses an interactive system of pictures on cards to encourage the person with dementia to express choices and preferences and respond to questions by pointing to a card. Requesting a speech and language therapy referral may be helpful if the family wanted to set up this system. Timing would appear to be important, as once a person's dementia symptoms become too advanced, it may be difficult to introduce this system for the first time.

From what I have seen happening in families, it can be extremely distressing and challenging for them to witness the loss of verbal communication in their loved one. This is one aspect of a person that makes them who they are. I would encourage families to see the changes simply as their loved one now communicating differently and to move with them on their journey.

15

Planning Namaste Care Sessions

As I'm sure has already become obvious, it is not possible to give precise, step-by-step instructions about how to deliver a Namaste Care session, as they will all be different depending on the needs of the person living with dementia. The personality, intention and skill set of the person giving Namaste Care will also colour the intervention, as will the timing and many other influences. Therefore, this chapter will provide broad guidance to consider when planning a Namaste Care session, in the hope that ideas for the content of sessions has already been covered in previous chapters.

As I began to think about this chapter, an acronym began to form in my mind when I was looking at headings to convey the main points, and that is P-E-G-A-S-U-S:

Preparation

Environment

Greeting

Assessment

Senses

Understanding

Simplicity

So let's look at each of these elements, most of which are common sense, but which work together to provide a loose structure that we can follow when planning a Namaste Care session.

Preparation

Probably the most obvious point, but it is important to ensure you have prepared what you need at the beginning of the session. Once you have connected with the person living with dementia, it is better to keep any comings and goings to get resources to a minimum to avoid added confusion, so ensuring you have everything that you plan to use easily to hand is very useful. In care home settings, where there is the luxury of an allocated Namaste Room, all resources can be kept close at hand. But in situations where there is not a dedicated Namaste Room, use of a wheeled trolley or individual drawstring bags holding supplies can allow things to be brought to the person, wherever they are.

Making sure you have a means to play music to hand, and that the music that the person likes is available easily, will keep things as smooth as possible.

It is also worth taking a moment to breathe deeply and prepare ourselves, prior to starting a session. Namaste Care is a beautiful and heart-warming intervention, but it can also be emotional and anxiety-provoking for the person giving the Namaste Care, especially when they first start. We are all our own worst critics, so being kind to yourself, and approaching the session with an open heart and a 'let's just try and see' attitude, will not see us go too far wrong.

Environment

Think about the intention of the session as your focus, which will usually be to provide gentle and relaxing stimulation. Does the person need to be positioned somewhere different in the room? If the person you are going to work with is usually positioned in front of the TV, for example, it may be better to move them if possible to another part of the room to signal something different is about to happen. They may need to be moved into a different chair, ideally one where they are well supported and slightly reclined with their feet up.

Does the lighting in the room need to be altered? Subdued lighting is relaxing, but too dark would not allow for good engagement in any activities, and older people often have poor eyesight, so this may need to be considered. If it's a beautiful, sunny spring day and the person has been sitting with the blinds closed, opening the blinds and moving them to be able to see a view outside is an easy way to provide orientation to the season and a change of scenery.

It is also worth thinking about the temperature of the room. A room that is too warm can make people sleepy, but equally older people can feel the cold more, so ensuring the room is warm but not hot will be helpful. Remember we will also be tucking the person in with a nice, cosy blanket, so we don't want them to overheat.

Ensuring minimal distractions is also a good way to support the needs of someone living with dementia. If there is a lot going on in the room around the person, they will find it very difficult to focus on the Namaste activity and they may well then disengage due to feeling overwhelmed.

Greeting

Greeting the person is our first opportunity to connect with them. Joyce Simard emphasises the importance of a positive, cheerful greeting, which values the person and acknowledges something about who they are. For example, a businessman who was brought up to be very formal with his manners and who likes to dress smartly might feel best met with a handshake and a comment about how dapper he looks today. Whereas someone who loves humour and hugs would be better met with a warm embrace and a funny comment.

This first exchange, if it is respectful and person-centred, can set the tone for the rest of the interaction. It can put the person at ease and encourage them to venture out of the closed world they can often retreat into when not stimulated.

Assessment

Assessment here does not mean a formal procedure – rather it is referring to an informal observation of the person's mood, level of pain or discomfort and level of alertness, and a general consideration of what their need may be at the present time.

For example, if a person living with dementia appeared sleepy and apathetic, it might not be a good idea to begin the session with a hand or foot massage, which would potentially make them even sleepier. In this situation it may be better to begin trying to stimulate their interest and wake them up. However, conversely, if a person was very agitated and restless, starting out with a gentle massage may be the thing to help them feel calmer and more able to engage in further interaction.

Non-verbal clues can be reliable indicators of mood, level of pain or potential discomfort. Indicators may well be individual; for example, I once worked with a man whose pain indicator was a lowered head, pale face, stillness and extreme quiet, when he was normally quite vocal, whereas for someone else the pain indicator might be crying out and agitation. This emphasises the importance of observation and getting to know the person well.

Pain

In terms of noticing whether the person is experiencing pain, again, as described earlier, this can be very individual. There are some formal pain assessment tools that can be used such as PAINAD and Doloplus2, which are based on observations of behaviour, but in a home-based situation there is not the need to assess a loved one formally for pain in this way. It is useful, however, to discuss pain, as, from experience, loved ones under-report pain in the person living with dementia. It is my opinion that this is partly because it is hard for them to think of their loved one being in pain, and partly because they may feel they are doing something wrong with their care.

Pain is defined by the International Association of Pain as 'an unpleasant sensory and emotional experience associated with actual or potential tissue damage, or described in terms of such damage'.

In end-of-life care, there is a concept of *total pain*, which I have heard staff from within our inpatient unit refer to and was first suggested by Dame Cicely Saunders. This describes a situation of physical, psychological, social and spiritual pain. They are all interconnected and influence one another. For example, if someone is in physical pain, then their mood will most likely be affected, and a person's mood will also influence how they experience physical pain. I think this is a useful way to think of the needs of someone in the advanced stages of dementia.

I will therefore address each of these aspects of total pain in order to encourage us to consider pain more widely.

Physical pain

The gold standard in pain assessment is self-assessment or self-reporting. Given the subjective nature of pain, having a person tell you themselves how and where they feel pain is obviously the most reliable way to assess pain. However, where someone is unable to report their pain verbally, we may need to look at non-verbal indicators of pain (see American Geriatrics Society Guidelines[1]). Some of these non-verbal signs are set out in Table 15.1.

---

1   https://geriatricpain.org/sites/geriatricpain.org/files/wysiwyg_uploads/ags_panel_on_ persistent_pain_in_older_persons.pdf

Table 15.1: Non-verbal indicators of physical pain

Facial expressions	Sad, frightened, frowning, wide-eyed, grimacing, eyes squeezed shut.
Vocalisations	Moans and groans, complaining, swearing, muttering, mumbling, whining, crying out.
Body movements	Pacing, fidgeting, muscle tension, jaw tight, fists clenched, repeatedly touching or rubbing a body part, knees pulled up, pushing people away (especially when being moved), hitting out in distress, changes to breathing.
Changes to how the person interacts	Needs more reassurance than normal, may try to draw attention to the pain or may become more withdrawn and avoid interaction.
Changes in activity patterns	Withdraws, less active or very restless, resists care.
Mood changes	Low mood, tearful, distressed, anxious, agitated, angry, aggressive.

As people become less active, their muscles and joints often become stiff and sore. You can help by encouraging gentle movements, either active (the person moves themselves) or passive (you gently move a part of the body for the person, being aware not to force it), and this is something that can be included in a Namaste Care session. A fun way to do this is through dance to the person's favourite music. This can be chair-based if needed, and a lovely way to dance as a couple is to have the person in the chair hold on to a large circle of elastic, and then you holding on to the other side, so that you can move together in time to the music.

Other physical pain can often easily be addressed with a regular dose of paracetamol; however, it is useful to have this discussion with a doctor who can prescribe appropriate pain relief for that person.

PSYCHOLOGICAL PAIN

Thinking about mood, Table 15.2 gives very general guidance, but bear in mind that individuals will differ in how they express things.

Table 15.2: Non-verbal indicators of mood

Low mood/depressed	Lethargy, sleepiness, pale skin, lack of energy, apathy, downcast eyes, loss of interest in food or overeating, tearful, staring blankly, decreased attempts to communicate, reluctance to make eye contact, slumped body posture.

Stressed/anxious/ angry	Agitation, fast and shallow breathing, pacing or tapping, sighing, distressed vocalisations, frowning, restless sleep, looking flushed and clammy, avoiding eye contact, tense body posture, resistance to care interventions, aggression.
Calm and content	Good eye contact, relaxed body posture, regular breathing, co-operative with care, responding to communication with others.

Addressing low mood may require anti-depressant medication in some cases, but can also be helped by increasing engagement with the person and keeping them more stimulated through Namaste Care interactions and meaningful occupation. I heard of a lady who was very down because she was unable to perform her usual family role of cooking and providing for the family. The family therefore devised simple tasks she could complete, such as stirring a pan or folding clothes, and her mood improved by feeling useful to the family once more.

With stress, anxiety and anger, lots of reassurance will help, as well as having a regular, predictable routine and using empathy to try to discover any causes of the stress. This can quickly address a difficult situation. Using calming room spritzes, surrounding the person with familiar objects and engaging them in Namaste Care will reduce stress levels naturally.

If there are ongoing concerns about mood, it may be worth discussing this with the doctor or the dementia specialist nurse involved in the person's care.

SOCIAL PAIN
As dementia progresses, it becomes an inherently socially isolating condition, but as discussed in Chapter 14, human beings (unless they have been profoundly traumatised) never lose the need for social connection. Loneliness has been shown to affect our health and wellbeing, and so connecting through Namaste Care will naturally address this need for social connection.

SPIRITUAL PAIN
Imagine if a devout Catholic has held a rosary whilst saying morning and evening prayers every day of their life from being a small child, and now they are separated from their rosary because it is not acknowledged as important to them when they have dementia. Similarly, think of a Muslim, whose day has been structured around a call to prayer since childhood, who is no longer able to express those deep spiritual beliefs in the same way. This must create

a deep sense of spiritual pain and separation from their sense of self. So thought must be given to how we can maintain these important aspects of religious life for people living with advanced dementia. The feel of a prayer mat, holding the rosary, religious music, scents associated with their beliefs and candles in the room, or whatever else makes sense to the person, are symbolic ways to represent their beliefs.

Spirituality is not merely about religion, however. It encompasses culture, beliefs and a sense of meaning that will be unique to each person. According to Speck (1988):

> A wider understanding of the word spiritual, as relating to the search for existential meaning within any given experience, allows us to consider spiritual needs and issues in the absence of any clear practice of religion or faith, but this does not mean they are separated from each other.

So, bringing the discussion clearly back to assessing spiritual pain, based on the Life Story of that person, we can know what has been important to them in their life in terms of beliefs and can seek to address this, but we should also focus on the here and now reality for that person. Viktor Frankl (1964) describes it this way:

> For the meaning of life differs from man to man, from day to day and from hour to hour. What matters, therefore, is not the meaning of life in general but rather the meaning of a person's life at a given moment.

What matters right now? The person living with advanced dementia may struggle to express the most basic needs, so think about it this way: they are not able to clearly process cognitively very well any more and are experiencing the world through physical sensations and emotions, so what does the person appear to be communicating? I'm thirsty? I'm lonely? I'm scared? I'm hungry? I'm bored? I'm cold or hot? A meaningful activity in this moment may only need to be as simple as holding the person's hand and reassuring them or getting them something to drink that they will enjoy.

Positioning/seating

The final area to consider under assessing current need is to look at the person's level of comfort with their seating. A wheelchair is not the best kind of seating for Namaste Care as there is little support and often the person is in a slumped position. Having the person in a chair that is reclined or with their feet up, and ensuring that their whole body is well supported, will allow them to relax and focus on the Namaste Care interaction. Also making sure they are not sitting in a cold draught, too near a radiator or with the sun in their eyes will ensure their comfort levels are considered.

Senses

We can give some forethought to how we might attempt to gently stimulate each sense throughout the session. This is explored in full in Chapter 12 and 13. All senses are important and can evoke pleasant memories, especially smell, taste and sound.

We can give consideration to how we use sound in a session as we prepare. As mentioned previously, it is better to not have any background noise as a distraction from your Namaste activities. This will allow us to use sound creatively and relationally throughout the session. First, let's think about how we use our own voice.

Whilst we can use our voice to explain things, comment on things and inform the person we are spending time with, it is easy for our own anxiety to lead us to chatter too much, and this in itself can become overwhelming to someone with advanced dementia. So it may be useful to think about pace of speech as well as of the session overall and slow that right down too. Loudness will vary depending on the person. Some people with hearing problems may need you to speak up, while others may be sensitive to sound and need you to use a quieter tone of voice.

We should not be uncomfortable with silences. It is very appropriate to have quiet moments, such as during massages or when listening to music. However, I would add a note of caution. I experimented recently with sitting next to someone with advanced dementia that I was visiting, listening to his favourite music and not speaking at all. I think this led to his losing all sense that I was there, and he fell asleep. I was sitting at the edges of his peripheral vision and in that moment I disappeared in his experience. Therefore, I concluded that we can keep a person anchored and aware of our presence, either with the use of our voice or with touch, or ensuring we are very visible to maintain the connection between us in a session.

Using music is discussed in more detail in Chapter 12. Having a playlist of the person's favourite music is a lovely way to honour who they are. Also having access to general relaxing music that could be useful if the person needs help to calm themselves is also a good idea. Giving thought to the appropriate volume levels for that person, as with the use of our voice, will also help to make the experience as person-centred as possible for the person.

Loving touch, I would say is the foundation for the relationship we are building or maintaining with the person, so thinking about appropriate and soothing touch such as a hand or foot massage, hair brushing and scalp massage, hand holding and hand over hand guidance will be an integral part of the session you are planning.

Understanding

A clinical supervisor once used a metaphor to describe the experience of empathy. She said it is like two people standing on opposite sides of a river. The problem I was having was that I was getting in that river right up to my neck and being overwhelmed by my experience of other people's feelings. With empathy, it is vital to keep ourselves okay as we do it. My supervisor said with a smile that it is fine to put my foot in the water to test the current or the temperature; I just don't need to go for a swim. Naomi Feil also talks about the need to keep centring ourselves as we work with someone with advanced dementia. Our feelings of compassion and emotion can become very strong.

All that being said, having empathy as a foundation for a Namaste Care session is vital, as we need at least to go some way to trying to understand what the person living with dementia might be experiencing from moment to moment. We do that by observing their non-verbal and verbal communication and using that to inform how we are approaching the session. In a sense then, the person living with dementia leads the session; we offer activities, but we respond and shape the session depending on how the person with dementia reacts.

Simplicity

The themes throughout a Namaste Care session are 'one thing at a time' and 'keep it simple'. Someone living with advanced dementia can't process multiple activities and cannot cope with a fast pace, so slow down and introduce one activity at a time. Someone *without* dementia can only really fully focus for 20 minutes at a time, and this will be much reduced in someone living with dementia, so think about building in pauses: activity–pause–activity–pause. The pauses don't need to be empty pauses, as they are still an opportunity to connect and engage, so an example might be something like this:

CASE STUDY – JOE

I warmly greet Joe, who is 83 and was a 'Teddy Boy' in the 1950s. Joe is already sitting comfortably and I cosy up next to him to look through an album of old photos his family has put together for him. We spend five or ten minutes looking at the old photos; Joe points to some and recognises himself in the pictures. I make observations of what I see in the photographs, such as what he is wearing, what his hairstyle was and who he is with.

We pause while I offer Joe another drink and I suggest we put on some 1950s music.

As we listen to the music, Joe begins to tap along with his hands and feet, so I move to sit in front of him and offer my hands to hold. Joe takes my hands and we do a kind of seated dance along with the music. I get lots of smiles from Joe, and at times he sings along to the music. I watch for signs that Joe is tiring.

We pause, I turn the music down a little while I offer Joe another drink, and I comment how he used to do his hair in a quiff with Brylcreem and dress up so fine. I offer to style his hair for him.

I spend time gently combing Joe's hair and then apply Brylcreem and style his hair into a 1950s quiff. I gently wash his face with a warm flannel, taking my time and complimenting him on how handsome he is. I let Joe look at himself in a mirror and then I apply some aftershave that has always been his favourite.

We pause while Joe has some more to drink and we share a snack of his favourite childhood sweets that I have managed to find – white chocolate mice. I change the music to more mellow jazz music, which Joe also likes.

Next I invite Joe to wash his hands in a bowl of warm, soapy water that I bring to him along with a towel. He has arthritis in his hands and the warm water soothes his stiff joints, so I let him bathe his hands for a while before carefully removing the bowl and encouraging him to dry his own hands. I then offer to massage his hands, and let him smell two or three massage waxes, watching for which one he appears to prefer. I then spend about ten minutes slowly massaging his hands. I am quieter as I do this to allow him to focus on the relaxing sensation of the massage.

We pause while I wash my hands, bring Joe a fresh drink and offer him some.

I ensure Joe is still comfortable, warm and relaxed and then I read some poetry to him related to life in the 1950s. One poem is about going to the cinema and one is about going to dances. Joe smiles and nods as I read, but he seems to be becoming sleepy.

I pause and prepare to end the session by telling Joe how much I've enjoyed spending time with him and that I am going to let him relax for a while and that I will be back again another day to visit.

As Joyce Simard says, it's not rocket science. It's not a clever, technical intervention. It's just love and genuine care.

In concluding this chapter I want to add a note about over-planning. It is difficult to provide an exact blueprint for how to carry out a Namaste Care session, and this chapter may lead people to over-think and over-plan. We need also to be open to the unexpected, to going off on a lovely tangent and exploring that, and to not getting the responses we might have hoped for. So, whilst we might approach the session with a loose plan and set of intentions, it is fine for it not to go to plan. Embrace this with gentle curiosity and enjoy the ride.

16

Key Learning Themes

(including a case study contribution from
Chris Hayday, Occupational Therapist and
volunteer at St Cuthbert's Hospice)

Over the course of the Namaste Care Project so far, we have learned a lot, and the way we do things is constantly evolving in response to volunteer and carer feedback. I am regularly approached now by professionals from around the country who would like to introduce Namaste Care into their services, and in this chapter I'd like to share some of the things we have learned.

So, how do we measure a smile? How do we quantify an improved quality of life for someone living with advanced dementia? This has proved to be a thorny issue for us. With funders requiring feedback and fellow professionals looking for 'evaluation measures', this was something we have had to try to engage with.

I started off the project by completing the QUALID measure when I first met someone with advanced dementia. This is an observational tool used to measure quality of life for dementia patients. What became quickly apparent, and I know is something that other projects have found, is that given that dementia is a progressive condition, the QUALID assessment will not show any improvements over time, but that this does not mean that the Namaste Care intervention is not improving the quality of life for the person.

What we then sought to do with the volunteers was to try to capture any differences from the beginning to the end of the session through observation noted on our session records (see Appendix). These consistently show in summary:

- Increased eye contact

- Increased attempts to communicate verbally or non-verbally

- Willingness to engage in eating and drinking

- More relaxed body posture

- Improved mood

Carers also report that the benefits continue after the visit has ended.

We were fortunate also to have Northumbria University involved in evaluating the pilot project. Led by Dr Sonia Dalkin, a realistic evaluation was carried out, which involved focus groups with volunteers and interviews with carers (Dalkin *et al.* 2018). The aim of the study was to develop explanatory programme theories detailing whether, how and under which circumstances Namaste Care works in the home setting.

Dr Dalkin and the team developed some theories based on the focus group feedback, which were further tested and refined through interviews with carers. The theories that proved to be *supported* by carer feedback were:

- Namaste Care volunteers are able to evoke emotional responses from the person living with dementia, leading to outcomes of relaxation, engagement and alertness.

- Namaste Care visits provide an opportunity for carers to have restorative time to themselves, knowing their loved one is in safe hands, thus providing short respite from caring duties.

- The volunteer and the person living with dementia develop a strong emotional connection, leading to the building of a friendship, which could suggest increased quality of life for both the person living with dementia and the volunteer.

But there were theories that were *unsupported* by the carer feedback:

- There was no evidence to show that carers felt increased 'hope' as a result of Namaste Care, given the context that their loved one will inevitably continue to decline.

- Families have not been routinely keen to engage in the Namaste Care activities themselves. (Although I know of exceptions, this is generally consistent with our experience.)

At the time of writing, Dr Dalkin is seeking publication for the research findings as a way to continue to build on and share good practice within the field of care. Reflecting briefly on the unsupported theories, I am not surprised by the first finding of no increase in hope, as the carers are witnessing firsthand the decline in function that dementia brings. The second finding will require further thought as part of the development of the project, as it would self-evidently be a benefit for family carers to engage in Namaste Care with their loved one. Anecdotally, carers have told me that the reason this does not come easily to them is that it is so far removed from their previous relationship with the person prior to dementia that they would find it very difficult to try to connect in this new way. However, as with new volunteers just starting out with visits, there may also be an issue of confidence and knowledge, so it could well be worth exploring how we deliver Namaste Care training to carers in an accessible and low-pressure way.

Friends and Family Test feedback

At least once a year, we give out our version of the NHS Friends and Family Test to gain feedback from families. Comments received so far:

> 'This is the only service I have seen that places the patients' and carers' emotional and social needs above their medical needs, which is hugely important and brings great relief. The care provider is also excellent.'

> 'A chance for my Dad (the primary caregiver) to leave the house for a break.' (*NB. This only happens when it is a staff member, not a volunteer, doing the visits.*)

> 'Given my Mum "a feminine touch" which we are unable to do.'

> 'Provided an extra lifeline of support and understanding.'

> 'Any respite or additional help is useful; as a main carer my having to cope 24/7 can be difficult especially when the patient is a spouse.'

> 'Gives respite/freedom to get on with other things.'

> 'Reassuring to know patient is in good hands.'

> 'Given me some time to myself.'

> 'Has helped improve the life of my wife by engaging with her on a one-to-one basis.'

> 'Has given me the opportunity to talk to someone who has some understanding of the issues facing a lone carer.'

'Very friendly and professional service.'

No negative comments have been received.

Case studies

Another way to share the learning being gained in the project is through case studies, so I thought it was important to include some case studies and 'magic moments' in this chapter, before going on to discuss some specific points of learning.

CASE STUDY – KEITH (BY CHRIS HAYDAY, NAMASTE CARE VOLUNTEER[1])

Background

This case study provides an insight into the practicalities and interactions of a series of Namaste Care sessions involving an older gentleman, Keith, with advanced vascular dementia, and Chris, a volunteer and author of the account. The context is unusual in that Keith and Theo, his wife of 60 years, both have dementia and live with their daughter Jenny, who maintains a family home for her parents and also sustains working from home while being supported with care tasks by visiting carers. The couple were visited together by two volunteers, Chris, who worked closely with Keith, and Lesley, whose attention was focused on Theo.

How we began...

At an initial meeting when both volunteers were introduced to the family by the Namaste Lead, Life Stories for Keith and Theo were outlined, principally by Jenny but with contributions from Theo, and there were also opportunities for questions to clarify certain points. This information was used as the basis to guide both Lesley and me through the first sessions as we began to get to know and understand our 'partners' and develop ideas. Keith had had an impressive and extensive career, firstly as a young professional footballer and then completing his national service

---

1   Chris Hayday has a background as an occupational therapist and volunteered for the Namaste Care Project while also studying for an MA in Dementia Studies, now completed. He currently works for an AgeUK Dementia Service and is hoping to further develop relevant activities and groups for people living with dementia alongside carers and volunteers.

in the Royal Air Force, before training and qualifying as a schoolteacher, eventually becoming a headmaster dedicated to his work with children. He had also been a member of a men's choir for many years.

...and the routine that followed

There was a clear structure to the Namaste Care sessions, which always included specific sensory-based interactions; however, each was different in how it evolved, being informed and developed through experience. Each of our visits began with an enthusiastic greeting, often reciprocated with a warm handshake, bright eyes and a broad smile from Keith. A sensory hand massage followed our welcome, which was important for me to gauge Keith's mood and energy level, as I could carefully watch his face and expressions. Some specific visual stimulation was included through familiar photographs or selected film clips informed by the Life Stories (and 'requests').

A core feature in the form of a tea break allowed some time to rest if needed and, importantly, maintain hydration. Occasionally we would bring something seasonal to share, and as the Namaste visits ran through from winter to spring this included some Easter biscuits and a pot of daffodils, adding to the range of sensory features. The tea break also naturally involved all four of us in some form of conversation and inevitably included Peg, the family dog, attracted by the biscuits.

At some point there was also some specific element of 'audio' introduced (poems that Jenny remembered her parents reading with her as a child, choral music, a popular song or dance music from Keith and Theo's younger years, or a nature soundtrack). On two memorable occasions, an additional tactile feature in the form of a leather football was included, which Keith was able to receive and pass back to me, with some surprisingly energetic co-ordination. This was accompanied by a quality recording of a football crowd (sourced from the British Library archives). Many of the audio/film clips were played on a tablet, which Keith could sometimes be supported to hold or, when unable, could be placed or held within sight or close earshot. This meaningful and relational stimulation sometimes had a transformative effect on Keith's responses as he would become animated and communicative and, although his words were mostly unintelligible, we would share a vocal exchange for a few minutes as I would mirror his speech.

The ending of each session was often focused on the shared use of a twiddle blanket as a winding-down routine, and Keith would often be tired or dozing at this point.

Keith's energy varied a lot between, and occasionally during, our visits. Sometimes he was in a deep sleep when we arrived and was not easy to rouse. In such cases Jenny's confident manner and firm touch alerted Keith to our presence and led to some, albeit reduced, mutually beneficial interaction.

Reflection

Much of what is regarded as good practice across dementia care is cited as person-centred care. While this is a good place to start, I think that the opportunities for valuable interactions through Namaste Care can go much further. Although the situation described above focuses on Keith, it was also clear that our relationship and the wider relationships between the four of us (and occasionally Jenny, as well as Peg) were valuable and shared by all. This confirms the concept of relationship-centred care in a practical care setting.

CASE STUDY – BRENDA

Brenda was referred to the Namaste Care Project by Sharron Tolman (Admiral Nurse), who had become involved with supporting Brenda's husband when he was under extreme stress and experiencing his own poor health issues. Brenda was matched with our Namaste Care volunteer Evelyn, and the friendship between them developed very quickly and naturally.

Brenda and Evelyn spent time looking through magazines together, but as visits progressed, Evelyn noticed that Brenda's concentration and ability to follow a magazine article had gone. She therefore tried out flash cards with pictures and single words to great success. A picture of a hen, for example, provoked recognition, and although Brenda's verbal communication was confused, she was able to convey that her father had kept hens and it led to some lovely reminiscence.

After Evelyn had been visiting for a short time, she asked me if it would be all right to take Brenda out for a walk, given that she was still fairly mobile. This was agreed with our insurers, as previously described, and turned out to be a really nice way for Brenda to still feel part of her community. On walks, she met her neighbours, noticed the changes in the plants in gardens with the seasons and was supported to call in to the local shop to buy something for herself.

Brenda also loves to be pampered and so enjoys having face cream applied and having her hair curled, which is how she used to wear her hair. One day after Evelyn had done her hair, her husband came into the room and exclaimed that she looked like a beauty queen. Brenda was over the moon and it became a lovely magic moment for the three of them.

Further reflections on learning from the project

Learning themes that seem particularly important to share are:

- Limiting numbers of visits versus open-ended visits

- Session records

- Volunteer drop-out after training

- Need for a support worker

- Supporting a move into a care home

- Supporting people with dementia on a hospital ward

- Preparing everyone involved for end of life

- Referral guidelines

- Partnership working

- Namaste Care in prisons

- Pressure of seeking ongoing funding

- The 'Potting Shed' Men's Group

Limiting numbers of visits versus open-ended visits

When I read and was so inspired by Joyce Simard's book, my thought at the beginning of the project would be that we would match a volunteer with someone living with dementia and this relationship would continue until the person with dementia passed away. During my first training day at St Joseph's Hospice in London, however, it was highlighted from a logistical point of view that this would mean there would potentially not be enough available volunteers for new referrals, as there was no 'throughput'. The recommendation was therefore to offer ten visits, review, then if appropriate offer another ten visits before ending. With a heavy heart, this was how we originally set out with the volunteer visits. I say heavy heart, because it felt very much like a 'head over heart' practical decision and one driven by organisational need and not what was right for the volunteer and the person with dementia.

Very early on once visits started, volunteers began raising the issue of ending within group supervision sessions: how we would manage it, how would it feel, and so on. The anticipation of ending a growing and blossoming friendship appeared to be causing concern for the volunteers. We debated in supervision sessions how to manage the ending by changing to fortnightly then monthly visits before ending. We then toyed with maintaining 'keeping in touch' visits monthly after the 20 sessions had ended.

The place we finally reached came about because I truly want to empower the volunteers to shape the project, and what they wanted was to continue visits until the person passed away and then to keep in touch less frequently with the family after the death. This process occurred through negotiation, discussion and debate, predominantly in group supervision, and we have arrived at a place that feels intuitively right for all concerned.

I recently carried out a review visit with a family to see how their visits were going, and the husband of the lady living with dementia said he would be devastated if the visits had to stop for some reason. He said he felt that it was important for his wife to have her 'girlie' time with her volunteer, but also that he found conversation with the volunteer so refreshing, given his wife is no longer able to have such conversations with him. I always remind families that volunteers are giving their own time and that their circumstances can change. It would not be wise to create dependency. However, families appreciate this and are realistic about it, but value the ongoing, consistent relationship so highly that this arrangement truly feels the best outcome for the volunteer, the person living with dementia and the family. The decision to provide ongoing visits creates a volunteer recruitment headache for me, but that still does not mean we shouldn't do it.

Session records

Volunteers have recently updated the session record, making a third version based on their experience of trying to capture what happens in Namaste Care sessions. Version two, which we had been using (see Appendix), was an attempt to capture which activities have been tried in the session, what responses occurred, any issues that could be discussed in supervision, and any feedback from the carer. Crucially, as a group we tried to capture whether there were any observable changes from the beginning to the end of the session, such as improved eye contact, increased attempts to communicate, any changes in posture and mood, etc.

This version two has been partially successful. It has allowed me to get an overview of what happens in sessions and to record a summary of this on the NHS record of the person living with dementia. However, as the volunteers have been using these forms, they have found them to be ineffective in capturing the subtleties that may happen throughout a session and tended to become repetitive. For example, there may be increased alertness midway through the session, but this may not last until the end, and so if the level of alertness at the end of the session was recorded, it may give a false impression that the session had not achieved any engagement with the person. Another example would be if the ending observation was closed eyes, which may indicate lack of interest; however, it could also mean that the person has relaxed as a result of a hand massage. The volunteers therefore re-worked the form, based on their experience, to attempt to make it simpler and quicker to use, and to easily track changes and patterns across the weeks. The updated version three is also available in the Appendix.

Volunteer drop-out after training

To date, we have trained over 60 people in Namaste Care, but only about a third of that number have gone on to volunteer. Part of that is explained by the fact that we have had professionals attend the training for their own skills and knowledge development, and we have had some people attend because they have a family member living with dementia and they wanted to better understand how to support them. However, there have been a significant number of people who have attended the training with the intention of volunteering, and by the end of the training have decided that this volunteer role is not for them.

This is of obvious concern to the smooth running of the project and is something we have sought to understand by course evaluations and follow-up contact after the training day. What seems to have emerged is the potential volunteer's surprise at the level of emotional closeness that I am describing as potentially developing between volunteer and the person living with dementia. This to me goes to the heart of what Dr Dalkin's research highlighted, in that there is something going on in visits that creates a deeper emotional connection than a standard social interaction, and that for some people, this can seem emotionally challenging.

I discussed this recently with the current active volunteers in volunteer supervision, as I wondered if I needed to change how I conveyed the relationship during the training day. The volunteers felt strongly that it should continue to be made very clear and explicit, given that it is the truth of what occurs in visits, and that if someone is scared by the prospect of this closeness, then this volunteer role is not for them anyway. It was also suggested that a volunteer could attend the training day to support me and to give their account of what it feels like to build this relationship and to hopefully soothe concerns in this regard. I think this is an excellent idea that we will action in future training.

Need for a support worker

As the numbers of referrals to our project steadily increased due to our promotional work, word of mouth between carers, and regular referrals from professionals, I began to get a little twitchy about always having enough volunteers available to meet demand. I began to take on more visits myself, but this inevitably pulled me away from other aspects of the project, such as administration and volunteer support.

When we applied for ongoing funding, it was therefore important to think about increasing the capacity of the project, and we included in the bid, as well as the continuation of my role, an additional 18 hours for a support worker. The idea is that a support worker could take on visits that may be more complex and could also fill a gap where there were no volunteers available. Alongside this, it will be important to continue the volunteer recruitment drive, but the role of support worker has given us some safety within the project to continue to meet the need as promptly as possible following receipt of a referral.

Gaining Big Lottery Reaching Communities funding in 2018 was a huge relief and enabled us to take these plans forward. We have been incredibly fortunate to employ Bev Cooke, who is extremely knowledgeable, caring and capable, and this takes our small hospice dementia team to three people, led by Lisa Howarth, Admiral Nurse. Hospices have traditionally struggled to meet the needs of people living with dementia, and so this highlights the determination of St Cuthbert's Hospice to continue to develop their dementia support services. Having an Admiral Nurse lead the team brings the added benefit of support from Dementia UK, who have been very interested in and supportive of the growth of Namaste Care in the UK.

Supporting a move into a care home

As we set up the project, the aim was to support people who are living at home with dementia. The idea was that people who were living in care homes would be supported already, as many care homes have activities co-ordinators, and I would assume have dementia training.

The reality of the situation was highlighted to us when one of the ladies we had been supporting went into a care home for respite as her condition worsened and her husband (who had his own health problems) began to struggle to cope. The Namaste volunteer, the Admiral Nurse and myself all visited when she was settling in to the care home and were a little dismayed to see her lost in this new environment. She was wandering the corridors between the two locked doors, apparently looking for a way out. The staff told me that she was refusing to go into her room, so I asked which room it was and took her to her room, where indeed she paused at the door. The radio was playing loudly through the television in her room, booming out Madonna's 'Material Girl'. I pointed out to the staff that this lady did not like Madonna. I asked that they either play gentle classical music or have no music at all, as she preferred quiet. They were also struggling to persuade her to eat and drink.

It became evident that a way we could extend our project was to support a transition into a care environment for someone we had been visiting at home, due to our knowledge of that person and their needs. This experience also highlights a training and development need within care homes, where there would be a real benefit to learning the Namaste Care approach. People with advanced dementia can't join in with the bingo games or the quiz. It will not be meaningful for them to sit in front of a TV screen watching daytime TV. They can however continue to interact and enjoy a positive quality of life if they are given time and attention.

Supporting people with dementia on a hospital ward

Picture this scenario, if you would. A four-bedded hospital room, with four women with dementia in bed. One of them is tending to wander, so a nurse has been allocated to stay in the room at all times. That nurse is sitting on a chair in the corner, with arms and legs tightly crossed and an extremely fed-up look on her face. I'm guessing that in her mind she thought there were a lot more better things she could be doing.

This was the scene we were greeted with when the lady described above went from care home to hospital due to her deteriorating condition. That nurse could have used the time she was there to engage with the patients. She could have talked to them, held their hand, played music, read to them, given them a massage. Instead her body language screamed 'I don't want to be here'. What a missed opportunity. If we view things from the point of view of the medical model, I'm sure all the ladies had their medication, had their personal care needs met, had their fluid intake monitored, and so on. What they were not receiving was social and emotional support and empathy. They were just anonymous people in beds.

St Joseph's Hospice in Hackney have expanded their Namaste Care Project to support people who are in hospital with dementia, and this experience has convinced us that we need to do the same. This extension to our project is still in the planning stages, but will hopefully involve a group of volunteers being based on a hospital ward and giving Namaste Care to any patient who comes in who is living with dementia (with consent from the patient and/or family). Nurses are incredibly busy and over-stretched, and I don't wish to sound critical of them at all – they do an amazing job in difficult circumstances; but, hopefully, we can role model some less medical ways to settle a person with dementia while they are on the ward.

Preparing everyone involved for end of life

We know logically that if we are supporting someone who is approaching the end of their life, we are going to have to deal with them dying. But as we all know, there is a big difference between knowing a thing and then experiencing it and feeling it.

Helping people prepare for the end-of-life phase of dementia has become something we have needed to improve on through the project. I have introduced this now into the Namaste Care training day, so that volunteers begin to think about it even before visits start and can reflect on whether they can commit to a relationship that will end potentially within the next year. It has also become a running theme in volunteer supervision to discuss changes that will begin to happen as symptoms progress. The Admiral Nurse role (for us Sharron Tolman and then Lisa Howarth) in attending the volunteer supervisions has been a vital source of information and guidance in this regard.

We are also very well placed to support the family through these changes by gentle explanations and encouraging them to think about what is best for the person as the end of life approaches. Where and how would the person like to die? A hospital is not the best place for death in my opinion, but many people with dementia end up dying there if there has not been a clear advanced plan agreed. Whether the right place is home, a care home or a hospice will depend very much on circumstances and family wishes, and thinking about it is not easy, but we can kindly and straightforwardly address this issue with compassion to prepare all concerned. I feel strongly about this issue, so the following chapter will discuss this in more detail.

Referral guidelines

At the beginning of the project, we did not create referral guidelines, other than that the service was for anyone living in the central Durham and Chester-le-Street area who was living at home with advanced dementia. As Lisa Howarth explains in Chapter 4, this led to some inappropriate referrals for people with mild-to-moderate dementia. One referral was for someone with a mild cognitive impairment who hadn't been told she had dementia, so I turn up talking about a service for people with advanced dementia and it was all a bit awkward. Much back-pedalling occurred, I offered to spend some time with her doing a Life Story, and both she and the family were left happy in the knowledge that, when the time came, the service was there for her.

It therefore became increasingly obvious that some professionals didn't have a clear idea about the intentions of the project. I believe they thought it was a bit like befriending. However, there are other services that provide befriender services, such as the Alzheimer's Society's 'Side by Side' project and Age UK's befriender services. I began a series of visits to our local community teams of nurses, occupational therapists, and so on, to explain the nature of the project and what advanced dementia means in the context of the project. We also developed some referral guidelines (see Appendix) to go along with the referral form. My concern about referral guidelines is that people will then be reluctant to refer in case they 'get it wrong' in terms of a person's stage of dementia progression, so we will monitor referral numbers going forward with this in mind.

Partnership working

From my time in a career working in social services, the voluntary sector, private organisations and NHS settings, I realise how much excellent work is going on that doesn't get shared. Organisations can become very insular and inflexible without listening to other ways of doing things and other points of view. My time at St Cuthbert's Hospice has been extremely positive from the point of view of meeting, networking, consulting with and working with other organisations. This means that services don't get unnecessarily duplicated, learning is shared, which can enable other organisations to set up Namaste Care services more quickly by being available for advice and consultation, and we can build a network of other services that we can refer families to. We really are stronger together. Namaste Care International can be an excellent facilitator of this network and I would recommend looking at their website (see Useful Resources).

Namaste Care in prisons

Obviously, within the prison population there is a small percentage of people living with dementia. Our local Alzheimer's Society branch have done an excellent job of training prisoners and staff in local prisons to become dementia friends, and there is evidence of prisoners becoming 'buddies' and watching out for their fellow prisoners with dementia. From a health care point of view there is a principle of equivalence, meaning that prisoners have the right to the same standard of health care as the rest of the population. However, nurses within prisons can't be experts in everything, and it has been identified as an area that could be improved on in our prisons.

We are therefore in preliminary talks with key professionals involved in prison health and social care to find out how we can support them. This will most likely involve training from the Admiral Nurse on dementia awareness, depression and delirium, and from me on using the principles of Namaste Care. I am aware this will necessarily generate ethical debates. There has already been the issue of the use of touch, which is so integral to Namaste Care, in a setting where the person may be a prolific sex offender. However, I believe that a fundamental principle of Namaste Care is non-judgement and compassion, and so it may be we can adapt and overcome these issues that staff will understandably have. It intrigues me to think that there may well be people in prison for serious crimes, who can't remember those crimes due to their dementia. Imagine that. Imagine waking up in a prison cell and not knowing why.

Pressure of seeking ongoing funding

Whereas Namaste Care in care home settings can become part of the daily routine and services offered, Namaste Care in the community requires funding in order to set up, organise, run and develop the service. Our service currently runs with my post as Namaste Lead at 25 hours and a support worker post at 18 hours. So wages, together with overheads, volunteer expenses, training, travel and project resources, all require a robust and reliable budget.

The Big Lottery funding over three years has been incredibly helpful in giving us some consistency. However, the lead-up to being granted that money was stressful, and funding applications took up a lot of project time. St Cuthbert's Hospice is very fortunate to have had the support of two talented volunteers who are very experienced in grant applications, Rosemary Harrison and Susan Penswick. They supported the project wonderfully and were really instrumental in putting the bids together. But not every organisation has a Rosemary and a Susan, and there is huge competition within the voluntary sector for the same pots of money. I believe that Namaste Care could potentially be a commissioned service by statutory funding sources (I would say that, wouldn't I?), but again there are huge strains on public funding, so it could come down to some organisations running this as an entirely volunteer-led service in order to get it started.

The 'Potting Shed' Men's Group

We find it more difficult to recruit male volunteers than we do female volunteers. Also, culturally in our area of North East England, with its 'pit village' mining history and industrial heritage, we have found some men with dementia a bit reluctant to accept things like hand massage. Bev Cooke therefore came up with the idea of creating a men's group, based on the idea of a 'Men's Shed'. This will be an efficient use of her time, as she could see more people than in individual visits. So we are developing this idea, whilst staying true to the sensory principles of Namaste Care. Ideas for activities have included:

- Participants bringing a packed lunch and flask, as they might if they were going to an allotment garden

- Sensory gardening

- Very simple woodwork tasks

- Reminiscence work, including plotting where they live on a map of Durham and pictures of recognisable local employers

- Music

- Hand care at the end of the session (gardeners have to look after their hands with moisturising creams – hand massage by another name!)

This group will not be suitable for everyone and will rely on the man being able to leave the house, but for those who can attend it will be interesting to see how this is received. It's a work in progress.

There is a lot of work ongoing in Durham City to make it a dementia-friendly city. As part of this we need to consider the needs of people with advanced dementia too and continue to promote greater awareness within our community. I am reminded of one of my favourite quotes:

> *If I am not for myself, who will be?*
> *If I am only for myself, what am I?*
> *If not now, when?*
> *(Rabbi Hillel, Ethics of the Fathers, 1:14)*

This was written two thousand years ago, but it remains as constant wisdom that I believe we should ask ourselves regularly on a personal, community and societal level.

17

End of Life

Joanne Atkinson (Head of Health Continuing
Workforce Development, Northumbria
University) and Dr Caroline Jeffery (GP and
Senior Lecturer, Northumbria University)

The good death is difficult to define; it is a dynamic concept, which evolves according to the moment in time, culture and societal forces (Cottrell and Duggleby 2016), and is significantly affected by the disease which will become the primary cause of death. As dementia is a progressive brain disease, patients and their families appreciate the trajectory from the outset.

Palliative care is a key component of care delivery, for people with dementia and their families. Palliative care is an approach that improves the quality of life of patients and their families who are facing problems associated with life-limiting illness. It prevents and relieves suffering through the early identification, correct assessment and treatment of pain and other problems, whether physical, psychosocial or spiritual. Assessing suffering involves taking care of issues beyond physical symptoms. Palliative care uses a team approach to support patients and their caregivers (World Health Organization 2015).

There can be confusion around the terms *palliative care* and *end-of-life care* – they are not mutually exclusive. It is imperative to recognise that patients and their families have the right to access high-quality palliative care and end-of-life care services. Such access will enable greater probability of exercising choice about their preferred place of care at the end of their life (National Council of Palliative Care 2010). End-of-life care services should support people approaching the end of their life to live as well as possible until their death.

While the patient has insight, this support should focus not only on the physical symptoms, which in dementia can be vast and varied (Sampson *et al.* 2006), but also on the psychological effect that losing your memory can have on the patient and their family. The physical symptoms are not limited to the disease process itself but also the effects of that process on the rest of the body. For example, a reduction in the ability to self-care, due to the dementia, may cause problems like dental abscesses through lack of teeth brushing and pressure sores through lack of movement. Forgetting medication may exacerbate other long-term conditions, and failure to recognise symptoms may result in delayed presentation at the GP's surgery with infections. All of this adds to the burden of the disease despite not being directly caused by the dementia itself. At the end of life, as with all disease processes, the care should not focus only on the disease process but also on all its effects, with a view to achieving comfort. The effects of dementia do not follow a predictable trajectory; therefore regular reviews of symptoms are important, never more so than at the end of life. In end-stage advanced dementia, there are a series of false dawns and false alarms. False dawns occur when the patient is deemed to be deteriorating but then becomes more wakeful and even responsive, giving the family false hope of more time. In contrast, false alarms occur when the patient has a critical deterioration (e.g. as a result of infection) which can be treated. The impact on the family of these false dawns and false alarms is great, as they have been living for years with the diagnosis of dementia and the inevitability of death; however, the unpredictable nature of dying with dementia is like living on a rollercoaster. The impact of this and the toll it takes on the patient's caregivers should not be underestimated, and it is important to support everyone involved.

As death approaches

Knowing the patient, understanding the person, following their wishes and providing individual care is a key component to deliver quality care at the end of life, enabling choice and adhering to wishes (Costello 2006; Froggatt *et al.* 2006), and is important for patients and their families after living with and dying from dementia. One of the challenges as death approaches is where the patient wants to die, their preferred place of care.

It is important to recognise that place of death is not simply about patient choice but also about the complexities of dying, environmental factors and availability of services (Constantini 2008). Nevertheless, an essential consideration for a good death is for people to be able to die in the place they want to (Seymour, French and Richardson 2010). In order for this to be achievable, the patient's choice and wishes must be discussed and captured so that all members of the professional team caring for the patient can make this achievable and can circumvent professional and societal barriers and demands that may stifle choice (Clarke and Seymour 2010; Cox *et al.* 2011). The challenge is to ensure a distinction is made between preferred place of care and preferred place of death (Agar *et al.* 2008). These can differ: for example, people may well want to be cared for in hospital; however, as death approaches, they may well then want to go home or to a hospice to die (Gerrard, Campbell and Munton 2011).

In order to ensure quality of care at the end of life, the principles of palliative care have to be embedded in all therapeutic relationships. Without a strong, functional and engaged multi-professional team, the patient and their family may be subjected to fragmented care delivery (Lee *et al.* 2015). The lasting effects of incomplete care can live long in the memory of the family left behind.

There are some key principles that are fundamental to the delivery of high-quality end-of-life care. First, the culture of care must be patient- and family-focused, delivered by a true multi-professional team with the requisite knowledge, skills and expertise to deliver effective symptom control, psychological support and adherence to a holistic philosophy. Second, the team must have strong leadership and management with a clear integration of clinical expertise (Lee *et al.* 2015). Third, as is so often the case at the end of life, in chronic disease there are issues related to access and equity of appropriate end-of-life care. This is common to all chronic diseases and impacts upon the timely delivery of care and recognition of need at the end of life (Atkinson and Quinn 2017). In addition, as people age there is a strong likelihood that alongside their dementia diagnosis there will also be multiple co-morbidities, which complicates how we deliver care and co-ordinate management of the patient journey (Reed, Clarke and Macfarlane 2012).

When considering the notion of the multi-professional team, it must be recognised that palliative care is the business of every health and social care professional in general terms. Specialist palliative care is required for a significant minority of patients – those who have complex symptoms and psychological difficulties. As we have discussed often for the dementia patient and their families, there are complex symptoms, so it is vitally important that the multi-professional team is harnessed for all of its strengths to provide the best-quality end-of-life care. Namaste Care contributes significantly to the quality of care for people with advanced dementia, reaching the end of their life through improving communication, delivering holistic care and promoting quality of life (Stacpoole *et al.* 2014).

The multi-professional team can be wide and varied; it may include, but not be limited to, nurses, doctors, physiotherapists, dieticians, social workers, consultants, district nurses and pharmacists. Communication between team members needs to be effective, timely and frequent to ensure that all members are aware of their role and how they can dovetail with each other to support each other and, moreover, the patient and their family. Thus they are able to work together to give clear information to the family, avoiding too many false dawns and false alarms. One of the key issues that causes significant impact on quality of care at the end of life is the fragmentation of services, so robust communication and integration are key in order to achieve good end-of-life care (Lee *et al.* 2015).

The priorities, as we change gear at the end of life, should include supporting the patient and their family and maximising symptom control. In terms of supporting the family, careful communication is important so that they understand that their loved one is reaching the end of their life; assumptions cannot be made that the family know that the end of life approaches, as they will have seen many times before a deterioration followed by a period of stability. As professionals, we can take for granted our knowledge and experience and forget that for the family this is their experience, and quite feasibly their only experience of caring for someone who is reaching the end of their life. At this time, therefore, we should be open with them, supportive, honest and compassionate.

Recognising dying

Recognising the last days or hours of a patient's life is difficult. There may well be physical and behavioural changes over the weeks and even months before death, and there will certainly be a gradual weakening and changes in appearance – the colour of the skin may change and become translucent, and they may have gaunt facial features and glazed eyes. There will be changes to physical functioning, more profound weakness, longer periods of sleep and changes to the voice and ways of communicating. As death approaches, changes in mental awareness (which in dementia is difficult to assess) and restlessness may become problematic. The patient's appetite may reduce and they may refuse food, a distressing symptom for the family and one that is common as part of the dementia disease process (Pinzen *et al.* 2013). This example alone highlights the difficult nature of recognising dying in the dementia patient, as food refusal may have been a feature of their illness for some time. Careful communication and continuity of care will help the professional team involved, together with the family, reach the conclusion that death approaches.

Symptom management should be as important at this stage in a person's life as at any other. The clear aim is to ensure comfort and minimise distress. Pain, agitation and shortness of breath are thought to be the most common symptoms in end-of-life dementia care (Hendricks *et al.* 2014), and these are also all common symptoms in patients dying from other illnesses. All symptoms should be treated effectively and proactively as with other disease processes. In many ways, caring for a patient dying from dementia is much like with any other illness. Our aim is to address their psychical, psychological and social needs. The added layer of complexity comes when the patient has lost their ability to communicate their wishes – difficult communication can mean that it is hard to establish the cause of the apparent distress in the patient. Communication of potential side-effects and capacity to decide upon a course of treatment are impaired in end-stage dementia but should not prevent good care. Capacity should not be presumed based on a diagnosis of dementia and will vary from situation to situation and patient to patient (Dickens *et al.* 2018).

Frank and open discussions early in the disease process can often help the caregiver at the end of life to be aware of the wishes of their loved one. Having clear discussions in the early stages of the illness before capacity begins to fade will help the grieving process for those left behind, knowing that they looked after their loved one as they would have liked. This should form part of the post-diagnosis package of care, which currently often has poor uptake by patients (Livingstone *et al.* 2017). This poor uptake could be a reflection of the difficulties the patient has in imagining their future self, and it could be linked to the common reluctance to accept the reality of the diagnosis.

Most people with dementia are over 65 years old; hence it is likely they have other co-morbidities, and this should not be forgotten during their end-of-life care. Consideration should be given to the impact of these conditions on their symptoms, remembering that they may not display symptoms in the same way, or be able to articulate these as clearly.

A lack of planning should not impede care, and addressing all symptoms in the patient's best interest is fundamental to care at the end of life. Significantly, studies suggest that most people choose to be at home to die (Higginson and Sengupta 2000); however, as death approaches, place of death and choices are ever changing, dependent on circumstances, changing condition and carer burden (Gott, Seymour and Bellamy 2004; Munday, Petrova and Dale 2009; Pollock 2015). Such a changing landscape has to be reflected in the discussions that enable patient preferences to be communicated; choices evolve, they can be blocked by professionals and by availability of services, and they can be communicated poorly and at inappropriate times (Munday *et al.* 2009). Ensuring a comfortable, peaceful, good death does not solely rely on forward planning; the professional team should have the experience to deal with the symptoms and situations that arise.

The dying process

As we have established, families may not be aware of the process of dying, and talking them through the process and the signs and symptoms they can expect to see may help reduce anxiety. Towards the end of life, patients will be increasingly sleepy and drifting in and out of consciousness, and this is a natural and peaceful part of death. Reduced oral intake and an inability to swallow are often distressing to the family; they should be reassured that keeping the patient's mouth moist and lips hydrated with lip balm are all that is needed.

Terminal restlessness can be very distressing for the family to witness; it is a symptom in its own right but also may be a sign of pain or discomfort. These symptoms should be explored to ensure that the patient is not too hot or cold and is comfortable. A patient's breathing pattern will alter; it may slow and stop for short periods before restarting. This again may be alarming for the family and needs careful explanation. In addition, and particularly distressing for the family, respiratory secretions make bubbly sounds, and whilst this can be controlled with medication, reassurance that this is not distressing to the patient may offer some comfort. Patients may appear pale and be cold and clammy. This is due to altered blood flow; the family should be reassured, and all symptoms and the associated management discussed with them. Human touch and contact will help calm the patient. Ensure spiritual needs are met whatever these may be.

Namaste Care plays an important part in the delivery of patient- and family-focused care at the end of life, offering a different means of expression and communication. Those professionals who know the patient and the family best should offer family support.

The grief process

Grieving for dementia patients is often different from grieving for those who have died from other illnesses. Often the person they knew and loved seems to have gone long before their death. So cruel is the disease that this can be years in advance of physical death. Grief therefore can come in stages, each time mourning for part of their loved one.

Several models have been applied to this process, each offering insight into the stages of the disease, from diagnosis and loss of normal activities to transitioning into a phase where more care is needed, increasing social isolation until eventual death. Whichever way grieving is considered, it is complex and a long journey for the patient and their carers.

Because of activities that the patient and family members can no longer do together, a memory they can no longer reflect on and laugh about, or a place they can no longer travel to, anticipatory grief increases and social death occurs (George 2010; Gott 2008). Time can be distressing as the person they knew is replaced by someone who at times is unrecognisable from the person they loved, who may even become violent and have a different personality entirely. The strain that this can place on a family and the patient's therapy team should not be underestimated. Caring for someone who is dying is a difficult task for families, regardless of the pathology behind the death, but in dementia this is heightened, as the person in front of them is not the person who they know, and this at times can feel like caring for a stranger, posing more guilt and stress on the family. In turn, once someone dies, there is often a feeling of relief, and this is a recognised and valid feeling but can often bring more guilt with it, making the grieving process long and difficult.

Bereavement counselling can pay a crucial role in helping at this time and over the forthcoming months and years. Increased emotional support before death can decrease the need for this after death occurs, and the family feeling valued and cared for throughout this process is a vital component of end-of-life care (Robinson, Hughes and Daley 2006).

18

Conclusion

As I sit reflecting on the conclusion of this book, I am mindful that all that I have written here is about to become even more real for me and my family, with my father's dementia diagnosis. I see him stubbornly and proudly trying to do the things he has always done, embarrassed at his struggles with word-finding and ability to write, and frustrated by his memory loss and growing reliance on others. All that he has been must feel to him like it is slipping away. Yet that very stubbornness is him. His feisty, determined, hard-working nature, that's him. We will need to find ways for him to continue to express himself and to feel loved as his dementia progresses.

What I have come to understand is that the close and special connection that builds between our volunteers and the people they visit is because Namaste Care is fundamentally relational. Martin Buber (1923/1937), the German philosopher, talks about 'I–thou' moments. and this reminds me of the 'magic moments' that Min Stacpoole of St Christopher's Hospice urges us to write down and capture.

Buber describes existence in two ways. The attitude of 'I' and 'it' has the 'it' as separate to us and as something we can use or experience (physical). However, where there is an 'I' and a 'thou' there is no sense of separation (spiritual). Buber proposes that humans find their meaningfulness in life through relationships. A person can enter an 'I–thou' relationship with another merely by being alongside them and directing positive thoughts towards that person or towards human relationships in general. There is a spark of connection, which is wordless and transpersonal.

It's an incredibly difficult concept to describe, but when I have these moments with Dorothy, we look into each other's eyes, there is a strong emotion of love, there are no words spoken, but the atmosphere feels electric and full of intense meaning. There is a sense of togetherness, like we don't need to speak anyway, we're just, well, together.

One moment shared like this came about when I was telling Dorothy that my daughter Holly had gone off to university and that I was missing her. I was reflecting that Dorothy had experienced this when her son left home, so I knew that she had felt what I was describing. She tried desperately to say something, and seeing her frustration I gently put my hand against her cheek and told her that I knew her well enough now to know the kinds of things she would say to me if she could. In response to my saying this, she visibly relaxed and she pressed her cheek into my hand and closed her eyes. I felt in that moment that she was comforting me in the only way she could. I was incredibly moved by this moment, but also worried that I had shared my negative emotion with someone I was meant to be cheering up. I talked to Sharron Tolman in supervision about this worry, and she reflected on what a normal thing it would be for a mother to talk about to another mother. In that moment we were sharing parts of ourselves in mutual support and understanding. She felt there was nothing more respectful, as I was truly treating Dorothy as an equal.

Another example is with a lady who I was visiting in her final weeks of life. Two days before she died, she had been mostly sleeping through the day, but when I put on some Glenn Miller music and started talking to her she opened her eyes and we had a full hour of non-verbal interaction. She enjoyed a hand massage, I brushed her hair, I wet her lips with orange-flavoured thickened juice and all the while she held my gaze intently. Then she reached out to me and pulled me to her for a hug, before wrapping her arm firmly round my arm and just lying there looking at me. What an intense and deep privilege it was to spend this time with her. I will never forget it.

I love the way that Teepa Snow describes the progression of dementia by comparing it to 'gems' with different characteristics. Her description for someone in the very advanced stages of dementia is that of a pearl. While we might see the outward rough, dirty oyster shell, inside there is a beautiful pearl, still pure and smooth. She describes it this way:

> While hidden like a pearl in an oyster shell, I still have moments when I become alert and responsive. I am near the end of my life. Moments of connection create a sense of wholeness and value between us. Use our time together not just to provide care, but to comfort and connect with me. (Snow 2018)

This 'gems' approach looks at what a person living with a dementia can still do, not what they can't. I would recommend reading about Teepa Snow's 'Positive Approach to Care' which encompasses a vast amount of advice and practical knowledge about how to approach care from the point of view of the person with dementia's needs (see teepasnow.com).

So, in conclusion to this book, I would invite you to create special moments. I would challenge you not to allow a person living with dementia to retreat inwards and to enable them to live the life that they are capable of, if we were only willing to adapt how we approach them. This not only benefits their soul, it benefits our soul, because when that person passes away, we will know we did all we could to give them the best quality of life possible. There is nothing to lose with the Namaste Care approach and everything to gain.

Spread the love. *Namaste.*

Appendix – Downloadable Sheets

1. Namaste Care Project Referral Criteria Guidance

2. Namaste Care Massage Consent Form

3. Namaste Care Service Referral

4. Who Am I?

5. Namaste Care Session Record (version two)

6. Namaste Care Session Record Summary (version three)

7. Namaste Care Family Agreement

8. My Namaste Care

Namaste Care Project
Referral Criteria Guidance

Namaste Care was developed by Joyce Simard in the USA as an end-of-life programme for people living with advanced dementia. Whilst defining advanced dementia is quite difficult, given that individual symptoms differ and progression of symptoms can be so varied, the following criteria are intended to provide guidance on appropriate referrals for the community-based Namaste Care Project.

- The person living with dementia lives at home in the . . . . area.

- The person living with dementia is most likely in their last year of life.

- The person living with dementia is finding it more difficult to communicate verbally.

- They have become completely dependent on the support of others for activities of daily living.

- They would not now find it easy to leave the house or engage in group activities.

- They would benefit from a gentle, sensory approach, on a one-to-one basis by a trained volunteer, to enhance their wellbeing.

- The person with dementia and/or carer has consented to the referral and is aware that the carer needs to be present in the house during Namaste visits.

CONTACT DETAILS

Namaste Care Massage Consent Form

Hand massage (and where appropriate, foot massage) can be beneficial to people with advanced dementia by helping to relax tight, stiff limbs and joints and bringing overall relaxation, connection and wellbeing.

Our skilled and experienced volunteers would like to offer you this service as part of their Namaste volunteering role. As part of the Namaste volunteers' ongoing training and support, they may want to discuss their interaction with you at their regular supervision sessions to ensure you receive the best care.

If you would like to access this service we would appreciate your written consent and signature. This is to ensure that you are clear about what is being offered and that you feel happy about that.

The role of massage has been explained to me and I am happy to accept this service.

I am aware that if at any time I would like to stop the session I just need to indicate to the volunteer that I am ready for the session to end. I know that this will in no way affect my access to the Namaste service.

Community member signature (if able to sign): . . . .

Carer/relative/guardian signature: . . . .

Date . . . .

[Carer copy]

[File copy]

Namaste Care Service Referral

(For patients with **advanced** dementia living **at home with a family carer** in the . . . . area.)

Request for an assessment of suitability for Namaste Care for:

(*The patient/carer has consented to this referral*)

Patient name:	Date of birth:
Address: Postcode:	Telephone Home: Mobile:
NHS no.: GP name: GP address:	Main carer: Relationship to patient: Next of kin (if different): Relationship to patient:

Referrer name:	Referrer role:
Referrer contact no.:	Date of referral:
Referrer address:	

About the patient:
Diagnosis/type of dementia:
When was the condition diagnosed?
Summary of current level of functioning:
Any other services involved?
Are there any reasons why this patient should not have a gentle hand or foot massage?
Is there any information regarding safeguarding or risk that we need to be aware of, given that our staff member or volunteer will be alone working in the person's home?
Any additional information you feel would be useful?

Please send referral forms to:. . . . .

CONTACT DETAILS

Who Am I?

Ideally this should be filled in with as much input of the person with dementia as possible (i.e. straight after diagnosis). Otherwise family members can fill it in on behalf of the person with dementia, based on what they have been told by them about their early life.

What kind of person was your father?
What kind of person was your mother?
Who were you closest to in your family? Why?
What were the house rules when you were a child?
What did you need to do to make your parents smile or laugh?
What was your father's favourite advice to you? And your mother's?
What would be your motto in life?

Adapted from the 'Brief Script Questionnaire' (Stewart 1996).

Namaste Care Session Record

★

Patient code:	Date:	Duration:

Activity tried and key observations	Products/items used	Tick
Face cream applied		
Hands massaged		
Feet massaged		
Fingernails filed		
Hair brushed/styled		
Snack offered		
Beverage offered		
Movement encouraged/ range of motion		
Reading		
Music		
Seasonal scents/items		

Observations about responses and preferences:

Issues to raise in supervision:

Observations on level of engagement and wellbeing

Indicator	Beginning of session	End of session
Facial expression (Passive/grimacing/frowning/ frightened/smiling)		
Eye contact (Closed eyes/looking away/ vacant/little eye contact/good eye contact)		
Interest in communicating (Avoiding/listening/non-verbal response/unclear verbal response/ clear verbal response)		
Body posture (Restless/tense/slumped/relaxed/ jerky)		
Mood (Depressed/anxious/calm/angry/ happy)		

Carer response to feedback about the session:

Any notable/significant responses to capture ('magic moments'):

Namaste Care Session
Record Summary

★

Visitor_____   Patient Number/ Initials _____

Date	Mood at Start	Smiled	Laughed	Spoke	Eye Contact	Ate/ Drank	Teary/ Sad	Calm	Agitated	Mood at End
Notes on this visit: (e.g. activities, moods, issues to discuss in supervision)										
Notes on this visit: (e.g. activities, moods, issues to discuss in supervision)										
Notes on this visit: (e.g. activities, moods, issues to discuss in supervision)										
Notes on this visit: (e.g. activities, moods, issues to discuss in supervision)										
Notes on this visit: (e.g. activities, moods, issues to discuss in supervision)										
Notes on this visit: (e.g. activities, moods, issues to discuss in supervision)										
Notes on this visit: (e.g. activities, moods, issues to discuss in supervision)										

Namaste Care Family Agreement

Namaste Care volunteer responsibilities:

- To arrange regular visits, up to 2 hours per week.
- To raise any issues of concern with the carer and the Namaste Lead to ensure the patient needs are met.
- To record session outcomes in order to monitor the effectiveness of providing Namaste Care.
- To inform the Namaste Lead as soon as possible if they are not able to attend a planned session so that the family can be informed.
- To respect the confidentiality of the patient and family.
- To involve the family/carers in learning Namaste Care and to feed back at the end of each visit.

Family/carer responsibilities:

- To be present during the Namaste Care visit.
- To ensure that supplies necessary for Namaste Care are provided.
- To inform the Namaste Lead as soon as possible if the patient is unwell and unable to participate in the session so that the volunteer can be informed.
- To respect the limits of the Namaste visit and not to ask the volunteer to do anything that is beyond the scope of the Namaste visit.

Namaste Lead responsibilities:

- Ensure Namaste volunteers are trained and well supervised.
- To be a point of contact between volunteers and families/carers.
- To manage communication between the volunteer and family/carers so that neither party need have the personal contact details of the other, unless this is agreed.
- To monitor progress and help to address any issues which arise.

Volunteer signature:	Carer signature:	Namaste Lead signature:

Date: . . . .

My Namaste Care

Include at least one photo that sums up who the person is.

'This is me'

I prefer to be called . . . .

My history	
I was born and grew up in…	
Places significant or special to me	
'Home' to me is…	
Things I remember most about my childhood	
My fondest memories	
The significant people in my life then were…	
Things that have happened in my life which are important to me	

Work and interests	
I worked as/my roles in life were…	
What my work/roles in life mean to me	
My interests	
My favourite things	
Pets	
Music I like	
Things I like about the seasons	
Smells I like	
Smells that may bring back bad memories	

My life now	
Who is important to me now	
Things I need help with	
Important routines	

Things I need to help me communicate	
Things that are important about my appearance	
Things that may worry or upset me	
Things that relax me and give me comfort	
Food and drink I enjoy	
What matters to me	

Physical/medical needs to be aware of:

My spiritual/religious beliefs:

This information was gathered together by: . . . .

Date: . . . .

References

Agar, M. *et al.* (2008) 'Preference for place of care and death in palliative care: Are these different questions?' *Palliative Medicine 22*, 7, 787–795.

Alzheimer's Research UK (2015) *Dementia in the Family: The Impact on Carers.* Cambridge: Alzheimer's Research UK. Available at https://alzheimersresearchuk.org/wp-content/uploads/2015/12/Dementia-in-the-Family-The-impact-on-carers.pdf

Alzheimer's Society (2014) 'Dementia UK: Update.' Available at www.alzheimers.org.uk/about-us/policy-and-influencing/dementia-uk-report

Alzheimers.net (2017, 13 March) 'How sensory stimulation can help Alzheimer's' [Blog post]. Available at www.alzheimers.net/2014-01-23/sensory-stimulation-alzheimers-patients

Arcand, M. *et al.* (2009) 'Educating nursing home staff about the progression of dementia and the comfort care option: Impact on family satisfaction with end-of-life care.' *Journal of the American Medical Directors Association 10*, 1, 50–55.

Atkinson, J. and Quinn, I. (2017) 'End of Life Care in Respiratory Disease.' In *Respiratory Disease.* London: CRC Press.

Ballard, C.G. *et al.* (2002) 'Aromatherapy as a safe and effective treatment for the management of agitation in severe dementia: the results of a double-blind, placebo-controlled trial with Melissa.' *Journal of Clinical Psychiatry 63*, 7, 553–558.

Beck, A.T. (1976) *Cognitive Therapy and the Emotional Disorders.* New York: International Universities Press.

Berne, E. (1961) *Transactional Analysis in Psychotherapy.* New York, NY: Grove Press.

Buber, M. (1937) *I and Thou (You).* London: Charles Scribner's Sons (English edition; original work published 1923).

Caldwell, P. (2005) *Finding You Finding Me: Using Intensive Interaction to Get in Touch with People Whose Severe Learning Disabilities Are Combined with Autistic Spectrum Disorder.* London: Jessica Kingsley Publishers.

Chenoweth, L. *et al.* (2009) 'Caring for Aged Dementia Care Resident Study (CADRES) of person-centred care, dementia-care mapping, and usual care in dementia: A cluster-randomised trial.' *The Lancet Neurology 8*, 317–325.

Clarke, A. and Seymour, J. (2010) '"At the foot of a very long ladder": Discussing the end of life with older people and informal caregivers.' *Journal of Pain and Symptom Management 40*, 6, 857–869.

Cohen-Mansfield, J. (2000) 'Nonpharmacological management of behavioral problems in persons with dementia: The TREA model.' *Alzheimer's Care Quarterly 1*, 4, 22–34.

Cohen-Mansfield, J. (2001) 'Nonpharmacological interventions for inappropriate behaviours in dementia: A review, summary and critique.' *American Journal of Geriatric Psychiatry 9*, 4, 361–381.

Constantini, M. (2008) 'Place of death: It is time for a change of gear' [Editorial]. *Palliative Medicine 22*, 7, 785–786.

Costello, J. (2006) 'Dying well: Nurses' experience of "good and bad" deaths in hospital.' *Journal of Clinical Nursing 20*, 13, 1824–1833.

Cottrell, L. and Duggleby, W. (2016) 'The "good death": An integrative literature review.' *Palliative and Supportive Care 6*, 1, 1–27.

Cox, K. *et al.* (2011) 'Is it recorded in the notes? Documentation of end of life care and preferred place to die: Discussion in the final weeks of life.' *BMC Palliative Care 10*, 1, 18–27.

Dalkin, S. *et al.* (2018) 'Namaste Care in the home setting: Developing initial realist explanatory theories and uncovering unintended outcomes.' Northumbria University, awaiting publication.

Dementia UK (2017a) *Delirium (Confusion): Understanding Changes in Behaviour in Dementia*. London: Dementia UK. Available at www.dementiauk.org/wp-content/uploads/2017/06/Delirium_final_single-pages2.compressed.pdf

Dementia UK (2017b) *Dementia UK Strategy 2017–2020*. Available at: www.dementiauk.org

Department of Health (2009) *Living Well with Dementia: A National Dementia Strategy*. London: HMSO. Available at www.gov.uk/government/publications/living-well-with-dementia-a-national-dementia-strategy

Department of Health (2015) *Prime Minister's Challenge on Dementia 2020*. London: Department of Health. Available at www.gov.uk/government/uploads/system/uploads/attachment_data/file/414344/pm-dementia2020.pdf

Dickens, M. *et al.* (2018) 'Understanding the conceptualisation of risk in the context of community based dementia care.' *Social Science & Medicine 208*, 72–79.

Ellis, M.P. and Astell, A.J. (2008) 'A Case Study of Adaptive Interaction: A New Approach to Communicating with People with Advanced Dementia.' In M.S. Zeedyk (ed.) *Promoting Social Interaction for Individuals with Communication Impairments*. London: Jessica Kingsley Publishers.

Ellis, M.P. and Astell, A.J. (2011) 'Adaptive Interaction: A new approach to communication.' *Journal of Dementia Care 19*, 3, 24–26.

Feil, N. and De Klerk-Rubin, V. (2012) *The Validation Breakthrough: Simple Techniques for Communicating with People with Alzheimer's Type Dementia*. Towson, MD: Health Professions Press.

Flanagan, N. (1995) 'The clinical use of aromatherapy in Alzheimer's patients.' *Alternative and Complementary Therapies 1*, 6, 377–380.

Frankl, V. (1964) *Man's Search for Meaning*. London: Hodder & Stoughton.

Froggatt, K.A. *et al.* (2006) 'End of life care in long term care settings for older people: A literature review.' *International Journal of Older People Nursing 1*, 45–50.

George, D.R. (2010) 'Overcoming the social death of dementia through language.' *The Lancet 376*, 9741, 586–587.

Gerhardt, S. (2004) *Why Love Matters: How Affection Shapes a Baby's Brain*. Hove: Routledge.

Gerrard, R., Campbell, J. and Munton, O. (2011) 'Achieving the preferred place of care for hospitalised patients at the end of life.' *Palliative Medicine 25*, 4, 333–336.

Gibson, L. *et al.* (2009) *The Power of Partnership: Palliative Care in Dementia*. London: National Council for Palliative Care.

Gold Standards Framework Centre (2016) 'The Gold Standards Framework proactive identification guidance.' Available at www.goldstandardsframework.org.uk/pig

Gott, M. (2008) 'At odds with the end of life care strategy.' *Nursing Older People 20*, 7, 24–27.

Gott, M., Seymour, J. and Bellamy, G. (2004) 'Older people's views about home as a place of care at the end of life.' *Palliative Medicine 18*, 5, 460–467.

Gridley, K. *et al.* (2015) *Life Story Work in Dementia Care.* York University Social Policy and Research Unit, Innovations in Dementia, Dementia UK, Life Story Network.

Hendricks, S.A., Smalbrugge, M. and Hertogh, C.M. (2014) 'Dying with Dementia: Symptoms, Treatments and Quality of Life in the last week of life.' *Journal of Pain and Symptom Management 47*, 4, 710–720.

Holmes, C., Hopkins, V., Hensford, C., McLaughlin, V., Wilkinson, D. and Rosenvinge, H. (2002) 'Lavender oil as a treatment for agitated behaviour in severe dementia: A placebo controlled study.' *International Journal of Geriatric Psychiatry 17*, 305–308.

Hospice UK (2015) *Hospice Enabled Dementia Care: The First Steps.* London: Hospice UK. Available at www.hospiceuk.org/what-we-offer/clinical-and-care-support/hospice-enabled-dementia-care

Hughes, J.C. (2011) *Alzheimer's and Other Dementias: The Facts.* Oxford: Oxford University Press.

Jackman, L. and Young, J. (2013) 'Exploring "unmet needs" in dementia care.' *Journal of Dementia Care 21*, 3, 32–34.

James, I.A. and Stephenson, M. (2007) 'Behaviour that challenges us: The Newcastle support model.' *Journal of Dementia Care 15*, 5, 19–22.

James, I.A. *et al.* (2006) 'Dealing with Challenging Behaviour through Analysis of Need: The Columbo Approach', in M. Marshall and K. Allan (eds.) *Walking not Wandering: Fresh Approaches to Understanding Dementia.* London: Hawker Publications.

Kabat-Zinn, J. (1996) *Full Catastrophe Living: How to Cope with Stress, Pain and Illness Using Mindfulness Meditation.* London: Piatkus.

Kitwood, T. (1997) *Dementia Reconsidered: The Person Comes First.* Milton Keynes: Open University Press.

Kong, E. *et al.* (2009) 'Nonpharmacological intervention for agitation in dementia: A systematic review and meta-analysis.' *Aging & Mental Health 13*, 4, 512–520.

Lee, R.P., Bamford, C., Exley, C. and Robinson, L. (2015) 'Expert views on the factors enabling good end of life care for people with dementia.' *BMC Palliative Care 14*, 32. doi:10.1186/s12904-015-0028-9

Livingston, G. *et al.* (2017) 'Dementia prevention, intervention and care.' *The Lancet 390*, 10113, 2673–2734.

Maslow, A.H. (1943) 'A theory of human motivation.' *Psychological Review 50*, 4, 370.

Mehrabian, A. (1971) *Silent Messages.* Belmont, CA: Wadsworth.

Middleton-Green, L., Chatterjee, J., Russell, S. and Downs, M. (2017) *End of Life Care for People with Dementia: A Person-Centred Approach.* London: Jessica Kingsley Publishers.

Mitchell, W. (2018) *Somebody I Used to Know.* London: Bloomsbury.

Moniz-Cook, E., Stokes, G. and Agar, S. (2003) 'Difficult behaviour and dementia in nursing homes: Five cases of psychosocial intervention.' *Clinical Psychology and Psychotherapy 10*, 3, 197–208.

Munday, D., Petrova, M. and Dale, J. (2009) 'Exploring preferences for place of death with terminally ill patients: Qualitative study of experiences of general practitioners and community nurses in England.' *British Medical Journal 338*, b2391.

National Council of Palliative Care (2010) *The End of Life Care Manifesto 2010.* London: NCPC.

Naumof, N. (2017, 22 May) 'Why Maslow's Hierarchy of Needs is dead wrong' [Blog post]. Available at www.naumof.com/single-post/2017/05/22/Why-Maslow's-Hierarchy-of-Needs-is-Dead-Wrong

NHS England (2014) *Sustainability and Transformation Plans (STPs).* London: NHS England. Available at www.england.nhs.uk/stps/view-stps

NICE (2006) *Dementia: Supporting People with Dementia and Their Carers in Health and Social Care*. Clinical Guideline (CG42). London: NICE.

NICE (2011) *End of Life Care for Adults*. Quality Standard 13 (last update March 2017). Available at http://nice.org.uk/guidance/QS13

NICE (2018) *Dementia: Assessment, Management and Support for People Living with Dementia and Their Carers*. Nice Guideline (NG97). London: NICE.

Norris, C.M. (2012) *The Complete Guide to Clinical Massage*. London: Bloomsbury.

Pearce, B. (1999) 'Using CMM, the co-ordinated management of meaning.' Available at www.pearceassociates.com/essays/documents/documents/84954_Glossary.pdf

Pinzen, L. *et al.* (2013) 'Dying with dementia: Symptom burden, quality of care and place of death.' *Deutsches Arzteblatt International 110*, 12, 195–202.

Pollock, K. (2015) 'Is home always the best and preferred place of death?' *British Medical Journal 351*, h4855.

Poole, M. *et al.* (2017) 'End of life care: A qualitative study comparing the views of people with dementia and family carers.' *Palliative Medicine 32*, 3, 631–642.

Reed, J., Clarke, C. and Macfarlane, A. (2012) *Nursing Older Adults*. Maidenhead: McGraw-Hill.

Reisberg, B. (1988) 'Functional Assessment Staging Test (FAST).' *Psychopharmacology Bulletin 26*, 653–655.

Reisberg, B., Ferns, S.H., de Leon, M.J. and Crook, T. (1982) 'The Global Deterioration Scale for assessment of primary degenerative dementia.' *American Journal of Psychiatry 139*, 1136–1139.

Robinson, L., Hughes, J. and Daley, S. (2006) 'End of life care and dementia.' *Reviews in Clinical Gerontology 15*, 2, 135–148.

Rolfe, G. (1996) *Closing the Theory–Practice Gap: A New Paradigm for Nursing*. Oxford: Butterworth-Heinemann.

Ross, V. (2011, 15 May) 'Numbers: The nervous system, from 268-mph signals to trillions of synapses.' *Discovery Magazine*. Available at http://discovermagazine.com/2011/mar/10-numbers-the-nervous-system

Sampson, E.L. *et al.* (2006) 'Differences in care received by patients with and without dementia who died during acute hospital admission: A retrospective case note study.' *Age and Ageing 35*, 187–189.

Seymour, J., French, J. and Richardson, E. (2010) 'Dying matters: Let's talk about it.' *British Medical Journal 31*, c4860.

Simard, J. (2013) *The End-of-Life Namaste Care Program for People with Dementia* (2nd edn). Towson, MD: Health Professions Press.

Snow, T. (2018) 'The GEMS: Brain change model.' Available at https://teepasnow.com/about/about-teepa-snow/the-gems-brain-change-model

Speck, P. (1988) *Being There: Pastoral Care in Times of Illness*. London: SPCK.

Stacpoole, M., Hockley, J., Thompsell, A., Simard, J. and Volicer, L. (2014) 'The Namaste Care programme can reduce behavioural symptoms in care home residents with advanced dementia.' *International Journal of Geriatric Psychiatry 30*, 7, 702–709.

Stacpoole, M., Thompsell, A. and Hockley, J. (2016) *Toolkit for Implementing the Namaste Care Programme for People with Advanced Dementia Living in Care Homes*. London: St Christopher's. Available at www.stchristophers.org.uk/wp-content/uploads/2016/03/Namaste-Care-Programme-Toolkit-06.04.2016.pdf

Stewart, I. (1996) *Developing Transactional Analysis Counselling*. London: Sage.

Stewart, I. and Joines, V. (2003) *TA Today: A New Introduction to Transactional Analysis*. Nottingham: Lifespace Publishing.

Tanner, L. (2017) *Embracing Touch in Dementia Care: A Person-Centred Approach to Touch and Relationships*. London: Jessica Kingsley Publishers.

Thompsell, A., Stacpoole, M. and Hockley, J. (2014) 'Namaste Care: The benefits and challenges.' *Journal of Dementia Care 2*, 2, 28–30.

Tondi, L., Ribani, L., Botazzi, M., Viscomi, G. and Vulcano, V. (2007) 'Validation therapy (VT) in nursing homes: A case study.' *Archives of Gerontology and Geriatrics 44*, 407–411.

van der Steen, J.T. *et al.* (2014) 'White paper defining optimal palliative care in older people with dementia: A Delphi study and recommendations from the European Association for Palliative Care.' *Palliative Medicine 28*, 3, 197–209.

Volicer, L. (2015) 'Loving touch: Treatment for rejection of care.' *Aging Science 3*, 3. doi:10.4172/2329-8847.1000e116

Walters, C. (1998) *Aromatherapy: An Illustrated Guide*. Shaftesbury: Element Books.

Wise, J. (2018, 17 March) 'The drugs don't work.' *New Scientist 237*, 3169, 26-27.

World Health Organization (2015) *Fact Sheet on Palliative Care*. WHO Fact Sheet No. 402. Geneva: WHO.

Young, J., Gilbertson, S. and Reid, J. (2017) 'Comfort care plans: A collaborative project.' *Journal of Dementia Care 25*, 6, 18–20.

Useful Resources

Organisations and helplines

The Alzheimer's Society
www.alzheimers.org.uk

National Dementia Helpline
0300 222 11 22

Dementia Carer Voices
www.alliance-scotland.org.uk/people-and-networks/dementia-carer-voices

Dementia UK
www.dementiauk.org

The Admiral Nurse Dementia Helpline
0800 888 6678
helpline@dementiauk.org

Namaste Care International
http://namastecareinternational.co.uk

Playlist for Life
www.playlistforlife.org.uk

Sporting Memories
www.sportingmemories.org.uk

Suppliers of massage products and room sprays

Aloe Forever
http://foreverliving.com

Base Formula
www.baseformula.com

Neal's Yard
www.nealsyardremedies.com

Songbird Naturals
www.songbirdnaturals.co.uk

Index